Liver Disorders

A CLEVELAND CLINIC GUIDE

Nizar N. Zein, M.D.,
and
Kevin M. Edwards, M.S.N., C.N.P.

Cleveland Clinic Press
Cleveland, Ohio

Liver Disorders

A CLEVELAND CLINIC GUIDE

Contact:
Cleveland Clinic Press
9500 Euclid Avenue NA32 / Cleveland, Ohio 44195
216-444-1155 / studerp@ccf.org
www.clevelandclinicpress.org

This book is not intended to replace personal medical care and supervision. There is no substitute for the experience and information that your doctor can provide. Rather, it is our hope that this book will provide additional information to help people understand the nature, diagnosis, and treatment of liver disorders.

Proper medical care always should be tailored to the individual patient. If you read something in this book that seems to conflict with your doctor's instructions, contact your doctor. Since each case is different, there may be good reasons for individual treatment to differ from the information presented in this book. If you have any questions about any treatment in this book, consult your doctor.

The patient names and cases used in this book are composites drawn from several sources.

Library of Congress Cataloging-in-Publication Data

Zein, Nizar N., 1963-
Liver disorders : a Cleveland Clinic guide / Nizar N. Zein and Kevin Edwards.
p. cm.

Includes index.

ISBN 978-1-59624-088-9

1. Liver – Diseases – Popular works. I. Edwards, Kevin (Kevin M.), 1970- II. Title.

RC845.Z45 2008   616.3'62 – dc22   2008005677

Cover and book design: J. Michael Myers
Illustrations: Beth A. Halasz, Cleveland Clinic Center for Medical Art and Photography
Illustrations on pages 95 and 97: Joe Pangrace, Cleveland Clinic Center for Medical Art and Photography
Illustration on page 98: Ross Papalardo, Cleveland Clinic Center for Medical Art and Photography

Dedication

To my mother, Khadijeh,
who gave me life and love,
and whose tenderness lives forever.

To my father, Naaman,
the rock of stability,
whose wisdom always showed me the way.

– N.Z.

To my family,
whose never-ending love and support
make everything possible.

– K.E.

Acknowledgments

As we complete this book, we would like to acknowledge the invaluable contributions of a master hepatologist, dear friend, and colleague.

Anthony Tavill, M.D., devoted countless hours of his personal and family time to scrutinizing every detail of each chapter for scientific accuracy and appropriate expression. Our great appreciation goes to Dr. Tavill for his dedicated effort that exceeded all expectations.

With sufficient funding for biomedical research, cure of liver diseases, including liver cancer, is within reach.

A special dedication of this book goes to the Mikati Foundation and its founders, Taha and Najib Mikati, for their commitment to saving and improving the lives of many through their support of medical research and advancements in knowledge.

It was once said:

"And there are those who give and know not pain in giving, nor do they seek joy, nor give with mindfulness of virtue;
"Through the hands of such as these God speaks, and from behind their eyes He smiles upon the earth."

– *The Prophet*, Kahlil Gibran, 1923

CONTENTS

Foreword

Those of us whose memories reach back to the practice of hepatology (the clinical science of the liver in particular) in the second half of the 20th century will recall the excitement that surrounded the discovery of the causes of many hitherto elusive liver diseases. At the time, this excitement was tempered by frustration over the lack of available treatments. That era has fortunately given way to the burgeoning of many effective therapies for a whole range of liver ailments. Furthermore, the desperation that we, our patients, and their families often felt in those days about diagnoses of end-stage liver disease has now been replaced with hope and optimism, thanks to the advent of successful liver transplantation.

It is therefore timely and appropriate to have available a concise, accessible source of information that communicates some of this excitement to our patients and their families. Often the time con-straints imposed on the modern office consultation leave many patients with questions unanswered. The liver is a unique, complex organ with many functions. It is not surprising, therefore, that patients are shocked and bewildered by diagnoses of serious liver conditions. Many are left with the impression that severely compromised life expectancy and quality of life are inevitable. Most commonly these conclusions are not justified, but have arisen because health-care providers have not taken sufficient care and time to allay the concerns of patients through explanation and clarification of all the issues involved in the consultation. Responsibility for this is ours.

This is why this small book is such a useful contribution to our patients' care and well-being. Written by an experienced, accom-plished liver specialist and a nurse practitioner dedicated solely to the care of liver patients, this book covers the entire expanse of liver diseases.

Having spent a significant portion of my career in the education of medical students, residents, and subspecialty trainees, I have come to realize that there is no concept in the biomedical sciences too complex to be communicated in simple, understandable language to the lay public. Dr. Zein and Mr. Edwards have accomplished such a task with skill in this brief but comprehensive book. Their case illustrations are enlightening, while their explanations of disease processes and terminology, diagnostic tests and available treatments are clear, concise, and accessible to all. They have provided the liver-disease patient with answers to most questions – answers that should allay many concerns arising from lack of understanding of the bewildering array of laboratory and imaging tests to which patients are subjected. Recognizing that good nutrition, psychological and spiritual support, and environmental protection play important roles in maintaining liver health, the authors have made many references to preventive measures and the promotion of liver health. Their book should be of immense value to patients, their families, and the public at large as we pursue the ultimate 21st century goal of preventing and curing all liver diseases.

Anthony S. Tavill, M.D., F.A.C.P., F.R.C.P., F.A.C.G.
Consultant Hepatologist, Cleveland Clinic Foundation
Professor of Medicine and Nutrition
Case Western Reserve University, Cleveland, Ohio

Introduction

Health is an ongoing public preoccupation nowadays. Every magazine we pick up, every newscast, even the home page when we power up our computers, seems to bring at least one health story to our attention.

And we love it: *The Biggest Loser* is a runaway television hit, nutritional supplements are a billion-dollar business, and thousands of people "Race for the Cure" each year to raise money for breast-cancer research. Health, it seems, is the new national pastime.

Yet we rarely hear people talk about the unsung hero of our bodies, the organ that fires us up, keeps us pure (in a manner of speaking), and keeps other bodily systems in balance – the liver.

If you're reading this book, chances are that you've been diagnosed with a liver disease, you suspect you have a liver-related illness, or someone you care about has a liver ailment. Like most people, though, you probably don't know much about this all-important organ or how to keep it from becoming fatty or hardened with scars. It's almost certain that you've never given much thought to maintaining it.

This book aims to change that. Think of the liver as a miniature sun, with all the body's "planets" – the heart, brain, circulatory system, kidneys, reproductive organs – revolving around it and depending upon it. That's how vital the liver is to us. If the liver's function is diminished in any way, our other organs and systems won't function well, either.

It's understandable that since the liver has so much responsibility for keeping us healthy, there are so many things that can go wrong with it. This book will take you through the possibilities and give you the most up-to-date information on how you, your family, and medical science can deal with those ailments. You will learn about common and uncommon symptoms of liver malfunctions, related conditions, how they all are treated, and what you can expect after treatment is completed.

So many questions arise. Is this condition contagious? Am I doomed if my skin has a yellow tint? Will everything break down? Will I need a liver transplant? You'll find answers to all your questions in these pages.

But the most important job this book can do is to show you that most liver diseases are avoidable and almost all are treatable and probably curable. Even liver cancer now is regarded as a "curable disease," and that's really what this book is about: your liver's *health*, and how to maintain that health into old age.

The health of your liver is key to your future. And as with many other aspects of the years ahead, you are in charge.

Chapter 1

The Amazing Liver

The liver, the body's largest organ, has fascinated humanity for centuries. As early as 3000 B.C., the Mesopotamians used clay models of sheep livers in worship, and the relationship between ascites (an accumulation of fluid in the abdominal cavity) and liver disease was suspected around 1600 B.C.

A thousand years later, Hippocrates studied yellow bile, black bile, and phlegm to devise his theories of liver disease, and he made note of cirrhosis and jaundice with delirium, among other disorders.

Philosophers entered the conversation in the 4th century B.C., when Plato and Aristotle studied the liver's function. Believing that a vein led from the liver to the right arm, Aristotle concluded that bleeding veins in the right arm would relieve pain in the liver. In the 3rd century B.C., Herophilus of Alexandria, a contemporary of Euclid, gave the first true description of a human liver, but it would be another 300 years before Cicero recorded the liver's role in bile secretion and the production of blood and urine.

In spite of these early discoveries, the liver's true nature would continue to be explored and argued until modern times. Select liver diseases were pinpointed and described by the 2nd century A.D., but not until the 11th century were the different causes of jaundice discovered by Avicenna, the famous Persian physician and scientist who wrote *The Canon of Medicine*. In 1654, British physician Francis Glisson published a landmark paper on the anatomy of the liver; 10 years later, Swiss pathologist Johann Jakob Wepfer discovered the lobed structure of a pig's liver.

In 1721, Dutch physician Herman Boerhaave finally connected hepatitis-caused jaundice to obstruction of the bile ducts, and in 1725, Italian physician Giovanni Battista Bianchi published the first comprehensive text on liver diseases. From there, progress came at a rapid pace. Studies of cirrhosis, liver cancer, and the causes of jaundice were published in 1761; Scottish physician Matthew Baillie linked alcoholism and cirrhosis in 1793 (in a groundbreaking book that was the first to introduce pathology as an independent science and the first to discuss organ systems methodically); in 1812, French physician Gaspard Laurent Bayle wrote the first paper on liver cancer of the modern age; and in 1819, René Théophile Hyacinthe Laennec coined the term *cirrhose* (in English, "cirrhosis").

A HARD WORKER

The liver performs more than 500 functions to keep our bodies working efficiently. Without a liver, our blood would be clogged with fats, glucose, and amino acids. Our bodies would have no defense against infections, no way to eliminate the drugs and toxins we consume, and no mechanism for processing digested food from the intestine. Our livers produce bile, store iron and vitamins, break down food and turn it into energy, produce and regulate many of our hormones (including sex hormones), and produce enzymes and proteins that heal our wounds and clot our blood.

That's a lot to expect from one organ. It's no wonder that scientists didn't know what to make of it when something went wrong. In the 19th century, an engorged or swollen liver was known as "congested liver" and thought to be caused by emotional disturbances, overeating, sedentary habits, and menopause. In the same era, other doctors were studying "corset liver" or "tight-laced liver," believed to be caused by the wearing of tight corsets or belts, a condition blamed for "dyspeptic" symptoms and abdominal pain. Treatment included bowel evacuation and bandaging the abdomen with elastic.

Those early researchers weren't entirely wrong. Today we know that this wedge-shaped organ, located in the upper right quadrant of the abdomen, is susceptible to many more influences than tight clothing. The liver is the recipient of every substance we ingest, from cigarette smoke to toothpaste to key lime pie – even materials we take in through the skin, including pollution and sunscreen.

Blood feeds the liver through the portal vein and hepatic artery (the word "hepatic" means "liver"), and exits through the hepatic vein. The organ is crisscrossed with a dense network of smaller blood vessels and bile ducts. Bile is a greenish, bitter, salty mixture that carries toxins out of the liver and digests fats. It is produced in liver cells (hepatocytes) and is released into the duodenum, or small intestine, where it helps digestion. It's stored in the gallbladder until we eat a fatty food; then the gallbladder receives the signal to squirt its content of bile into the intestines through the bile ducts to help break down the fats.

We think of bile as yellowish-green because of its bilirubin, a waste product of old red blood cells. When the liver is diseased, the bilirubin level rises, causing the yellowish tone in the skin and eyes that we recognize as jaundice.

Liver disorders have even entered the popular culture. Most readers will remember the controversial case of pro baseball legend Mickey Mantle, who had cirrhosis caused by years of alcohol abuse along with hepatitis C, possibly linked to a blood transfusion received during a knee surgery. During surgery for a liver transplant, doctors discovered that Mantle's liver also was cancerous; they successfully transplanted his liver, but Mantle died two months later from the cancer.

Mickey Mantle wasn't the only celebrity with liver disease. Singer John Phillips of the 1960s group the Mamas & the Papas underwent a liver transplant in 1992, but died in 2001 of heart failure. The late daredevil Evel Knievel contracted hepatitis from a blood transfusion; he received a new liver in 1999. And singer David Crosby, of Crosby, Stills, Nash & Young, was almost as famous for his drug and alcohol abuse as for his music. His 1994 liver transplant prompted public debate over liver-transplant ethics.

HEPATITIS C AND THE RICH AND FAMOUS

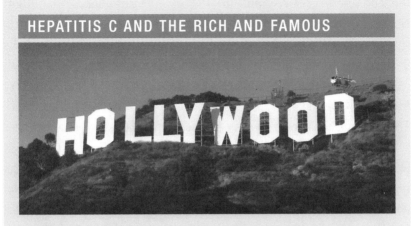

These are just a few of the well-known personalities who have contracted liver disease:

- Pamela Anderson, the onetime star of *Baywatch*
- Country singer and onetime nurse Naomi Judd
- Dusty Hill, bassist with the band ZZ Top
- Chuck Negron, former lead singer with the singing group Three Dog Night
- Phil Lesh, founding member of the 1960s rock group the Grateful Dead
- Singer Freddy Fender
- Bluesman Willie Dixon
- Steven Tyler, lead singer of the rock group Aerosmith
- Actor Larry Hagman, who underwent a liver transplant in 1995
- Porn star Linda Lovelace, who received a liver transplant in 1987
- Ken Kesey, author of *One Flew Over the Cuckoo's Nest*, who died of liver cancer
- Allen Ginsberg, poet laureate of the "Beat Generation," who died of liver cancer
- Anita Roddick, founder of the Body Shop (an international chain selling beauty and skin-care products), who died of cirrhosis in September 2007, after years of fighting hepatitis C

THE LIVER AT WORK

Among its other functions, the liver serves as storage space for vitamins A, B$_{12}$, D, E, and K, as well as copper and iron. Because we have stores of these vitamins and minerals normally, it is relatively easy to overload the liver with them, causing liver damage. That's why even a person with a healthy liver should be cautious about taking supplements of vitamins and minerals. Iron, for instance, is harmful in people who have a genetic abnormality known as hemochromatosis, which causes them to absorb too much iron.

Vitamins A, D, E, and K (commonly referred to as "fat-soluble vitamins") can exist only in fatty solutions, so when a liver disease causes the bile flow to be interrupted, the body can't digest the fats it needs for absorbing these vitamins. That's a serious situation in the case of vitamin K, which we need on hand at all times to help the blood to clot. Another little-known function of the liver is its role in processing amino acids, which link together to form proteins, the primary component of muscle. Without a healthy liver, our bodies can't produce and maintain the muscles in our arms, legs, face, or even in our other organs, such as the heart.

The liver is involved in our energy levels as well, by storing extra glucose as a carbohydrate known as glycogen and releasing glucose into the blood when we need an energy boost. When the liver isn't functioning well, the liver isn't as efficient in regulating the blood's glucose levels.

The liver even affects our mental sharpness. When we eat animal proteins, the intestines produce harmful ammonia during digestion, and the liver is responsible for converting that ammonia into urea, a harmless substance that then travels to the kidneys and eventually is eliminated from the body. When the liver is diseased, the ammonia doesn't get converted but builds up in the blood and brain, causing a form of mental confusion called encephalopathy. (The exact mechanism of hepatic encephalopathy is quite complex, and not solely the result of a high ammonia level. Research is ongoing in this area.)

WHEN SOMETHING GOES WRONG

Pinpointing a liver disease is not a straightforward process, especially for the layperson, because so many symptoms of liver disorders are vague and most can signal scores of other illnesses. Fatigue, low-grade fever, and flulike symptoms (such as muscle and joint aches, headaches, nausea, and weakness) all are associated with a number of liver disorders, but they also can be symptoms of many ailments unrelated to the liver.

RAW OYSTERS AND LIVER DISEASE

When the heat of summer gives way to cooler fall days, oyster lovers are eager for their first taste of the plump, juicy shellfish. But if you have been diagnosed with a liver disease, beware. The same conditions that create those succulent treats also are perfect for a bacterium called *Vibrio vulnificus*, which thrives only in warm coastal waters where fine oysters are harvested. In most people, the infection would probably cause only tame symptoms such as stomachache, vomiting, and perhaps diarrhea. In patients with chronic liver disease, however, the *Vibrio* infection can kill.

Scientists are not sure why liver patients have such a bad reaction to *Vibrio*, but they believe it might be related to high levels of iron in liver patients' blood, blocking their white blood cells' infection-fighting abilities. The immune system in liver patients isn't up to the task of fighting off this particular bacterium. *Vibrios* are free to move into the bloodstream and multiply, overwhelming white blood cells and often causing the patient to suffer from septicemia (blood poisoning), a condition that only 50 percent of victims survive.

Oyster lovers can take heart, though, from the thought that they don't have to give up their favorite shellfish altogether. Oysters are perfectly safe, even for liver patients, if they are thoroughly cooked.

MODERN MILESTONES IN LIVER RESEARCH AND TREATMENT

1912: British physician Samuel Kinnear Wilson first describes the syndrome that will come to be known as "Wilson disease."

1944: Hepatic vein catheterization is first performed to measure blood pressure in in the liver.

1949: "Fatty cysts" in liver cells are discovered to be the antecedent condition of cirrhosis caused by alcohol.

1959: Two surgical teams in different cities perform liver transplants in dogs.

1963: A surgical team led by Dr. Thomas Starzl of Denver, Colorado, one of the surgeons who had transplanted dogs' livers in 1959, performed the first successful human liver transplant. (A decade later, Starzl's research would establish the importance of insulin in the liver's ability to regenerate.)

1992: Doctors at Cedars-Sinai Medical Center in Los Angeles transplant a pig's liver into a woman in an effort to keep her alive until a human liver could be found. She died several hours before she was to receive a new human liver.

A few signals do alert doctors to a liver problem, but many do not present themselves until much irreparable damage has already occurred. Jaundice, certainly, is a clear sign of possible liver disease. Encephalopathy, or mental confusion, could be a first signal of a liver disorder. Pruritus, or severe itching, is another symptom that would prompt a doctor to run liver tests, as it can be present in any liver disease in which cholestasis, or a blockage of bile flow, has occurred.

Pain or discomfort in the upper right quadrant of the abdomen can be linked to a number of ailments, but it often signals inflammation or distention of the liver. (The pain also could be caused by a stomach problem, such as an ulcer.) Ascites, or accumulated fluid in the abdomen, is associated with advanced liver disease.

CAN THE LIVER REGENERATE ITSELF?

Contrary to popular myth, the liver cannot regrow like a lilac bush that has been cut back. At least, not exactly.

If less than 60 percent of a liver has been cut away, the remaining organ can expand, filling its former space until it reaches its original weight, and the entire liver can function normally, provided that the remaining 40 percent was not heavily scarred. This is what happens in many liver transplants. A healthy, living organ donor will donate part of his or her liver, and both the original and transplanted portions will expand and function normally.

In contrast to a healthy liver that is surgically cut, an extensively scarred or cirrhotic liver would not regenerate if a section were cut out. In fact, the stress of the surgery would be likely to cause the liver to quit working properly and yellow jaundice to develop, and the abdomen would fill up with ascitic fluid. ◆

Chapter 2

Hepatitis, the New Epidemic

When Janelle took the required physical exam for her new job, she felt great. She was eager to begin her future as human resources director for a national foundation that funds special education programs. She was ready to start looking for a condo and planning her wedding, scheduled to take place in a year, just before her 39th birthday. So Janelle was puzzled when her doctor's office called and asked her to stop in for a consult. How could something be wrong, when she was so healthy? She was a vegetarian, took long walks every afternoon, and rarely drank alcohol. Janelle wasn't a health freak, but she loved feeling good, and living a balanced lifestyle kept her energy and spirits high.

The doctor's grim expression told Janelle that despite her diligent investment in her own good health, something bad had slipped through. When he announced that she had somehow contracted hepatitis C, she was floored. After lengthy probing, Janelle finally thought of one possibility: About 20 years earlier when she was attending college she had experimented with some drugs at the urging of a boyfriend. She had allowed him to inject her with "something" but was so turned off by the whole scene that she quit seeing him and never tried drugs again.

The doctor prescribed pegylated interferon and ribavirin, one of the few drug combinations found to be effective in treating hepatitis C. Fortunately, a liver biopsy revealed that Janelle's liver wasn't too badly damaged. There was no evidence of cirrhosis (scarring), and her prognosis was positive. She would be monitored frequently during treatment and there was a good chance that she could get rid of the virus. Her doctors told her that if she abstained from alcohol altogether and kept up her healthy lifestyle, there was a good chance that she might never develop cirrhosis.

THE ALPHABET OF HEPATITIS

Hepatitis is probably the most misunderstood liver disease. The term itself simply means inflammation of the liver. And it is occurring in epidemic numbers: According to the World Health Organization, hepatitis infects more than 500 million people worldwide and kills some 15,000 people in this country each year. It takes many forms, which often depend on what caused the disorder. Autoimmune hepatitis and alcoholic hepatitis will be discussed in later sections. In this chapter, we deal with "alphabet hepatitis," otherwise known as viral hepatitis, or hepatitis caused by a virus. Only this form of hepatitis may be transmitted to other humans.

This collection of hepatitis varieties is named by letters of the alphabet: hepatitis A, hepatitis B, and so on through hepatitis E. Often, patients also will hear doctors refer to their hepatitis as being acute, chronic, or fulminant. These categories refer to the length of time the liver is inflamed; acute hepatitis refers to inflammation that lasts six months or less, regardless of the cause, while lengthier inflammation is chronic hepatitis. It is possible for a patient to advance from acute to chronic hepatitis. Fulminant hepatitis is the most severe form of acute hepatitis, with jaundice, coagulopathy (the inability to clot blood), and encephalopathy (decreased consciousness or confusion) that occurs in only a few days. For these patients, liver failure and subsequent death can come within weeks, and a liver transplant may be the only solution.

Even transmission of the viruses that cause hepatitis differs among the various forms of the disease. While some can enter the body through the digestive system, others are received during sexual contact or through contaminated blood. As we explore the A-B-C-D's of hepatitis, we'll discuss the various ways the viruses are transmitted.

One way of determining which form of viral hepatitis a person might have contracted is based on a series of blood tests known as hepatitis serology. In these tests, doctors look for antigens (Ag), the viral invaders, and antibodies (Ab), the immune system's way of fighting antigens. Testing for specific antigens and antibodies that relate to the various forms of hepatitis will tell doctors whether the patient has been exposed to those viruses.

HEPATITIS A (HAV)

Before hepatitis A virus was identified in the early 1970s, the disease was referred to as infectious hepatitis because it could be so easily transmitted from one person to another. Fortunately, the HA virus causes only the short-lived acute hepatitis; after six months, any inflammation, symptoms, and abnormal LFT (liver function test) levels are resolved, and the liver will suffer no long-term damage.

Few people are aware that HAV is so widespread. It is estimated that about 135,000 individuals in the United States contract HAV every year and that nearly half of all American adults over the age of 50 have been infected!

Because HAV does not cause chronic liver disease and there is no possibility that cirrhosis or liver cancer will develop as a consequence of HAV, it is considered the least serious of the hepatitis viruses. Moreover, HAV is totally preventable with a vaccine.

While it lasts, however, HAV causes people to be seriously ill, and if they have been diagnosed with another liver disease, HAV can be a serious, even fatal, complication.

HAV usually is transmitted by oral-fecal transmission, otherwise known as the enteric route. The virus will enter the mouth, then travel to the digestive system and eventually enter the liver. The infected person is most contagious during the two weeks before any symptoms develop and for one week after, though many patients experience no symptoms at all. Not surprisingly, HAV is commonly seen in day-care centers, where toddlers are bound to be careless about bathroom hygiene. Long-stay facilities for the mentally disabled also see frequent cases of HAV. Direct person-to-person contact isn't necessary; the virus can be passed along in food touched by a person whose hands carry the virus.

People traveling to developing countries, where standards of sanitation and food preparation might not be as stringent as in the United States, should be especially careful.

Symptoms, if they are noticed at all, might be vague, such as fatigue, headache, nausea, and loss of appetite. Children are more likely to be asymptomatic than adults. Pruritus (itching) and jaundice, with its accompanying symptoms of urine the color of dark tea and stools having the appearance of light clay, are common among older adults. Those who become very ill might need complete rest for up to a month, and a few will need hospital care. Jaundice, however, seems to be the climax of HAV symptoms. Signs of the illness tend to fade once jaundice has appeared. In rare instances, HAV can cause liver failure requiring a liver transplant.

Unfortunately, no treatment exists for HAV per se, but it is important to treat the symptoms. Patients experiencing fatigue need to rest and try not to push themselves. All HAV patients need to drink plenty of fluids because dehydration can easily develop as a complication, especially if the patient has had diarrhea. The good news about HAV is that it is almost always a preventable disease if a person receives the proper vaccine series. The HAV vaccine series has been used extensively worldwide and has proved to be a safe and extremely effective vaccine.

HEPATITIS B (HBV) AND D (HDV, OR DELTA)

The first hepatitis virus to be discovered, hepatitis B (HBV) has infected an estimated 2 billion people worldwide. About 300 million are chronic carriers of the virus, including about 1.25 million Americans. HBV can be deadly; its complications kill about 1 million people every year, and it is the most prevalent cause of cirrhosis and liver cancer in the world, particularly in Africa and Southeast Asia.

Yet, people infected with HBV can lead fully normal lives. HBV is a virus found in saliva, blood, tears, breast milk, and other body fluids, though it is transferred between people only through blood and semen. Casual contact, such as hugging or shaking hands, will not spread the disease; in fact, not everyone infected with HBV is contagious. HBV can be contracted only through sexual contact, a blood exchange, or from a pregnant mother to her fetus – a method of transmission common in Africa and Asia.

Before 1975, blood and platelets collected from donors (during blood drives, for example), were not screened for HBV, so that transfusions once accounted for many cases of HBV in this country. Today, even though donated blood is tested for HBV, the virus can be transferred through a more subtle "blood exchange," such as when an infected person shares a razor or nail clippers, or exposes another person through a bleeding skin condition. Needles used for tattooing and acupuncture, too, can be contaminated with bits of blood infected with HBV. Persons diagnosed with hepatitis B need to take special care to cover any bleeding spots, and everyone should avoid contact with used needles. The HBV virus can live on an open surface such as that of a needle for up to a week.

In this country, it's more likely that HBV will be transmitted through sexual contact with an HBV carrier.

FROM MOTHER TO CHILD

Pregnant women in the United States are routinely screened for the HBV virus during their antenatal care, and most babies are immunized shortly after birth. When a mother does transfer chronic hepatitis B to her child, the scientific term for the process is "vertical transmission." This can be prevented by administration of the HBV vaccine and special gamma globulin to the newborn baby almost immediately after birth.

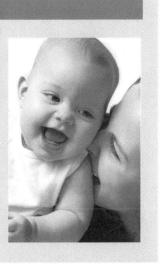

HEPATITIS B IMMUNIZATION

With hepatitis B, immunization is a key to prevention. HBV is nearly 100 percent preventable among people who have been vaccinated, and it is a disease that someday could be totally eliminated. For now, though, it's important for individuals at risk to take precautions. Health-care workers, anyone who received a blood transfusion before 1975, and anyone who lives with (or is sexually intimate with) an HBV-infected person are candidates for screening. In fact, it is recommended that sexually active homosexual men, intravenous drug users, dialysis patients, and anyone who has more than one sex partner within six months be screened for HBV. If these people are not immune, the vaccine series should be administered.

ACUTE HEPATITIS B

Acute hepatitis B, or HBV that lasts less than six months, is no longer prevalent in the United States, probably because of early vaccinations. It does occur, however, and its flulike symptoms resemble those of other hepatitis infections – fever, abdominal upset, nausea, decreased appetite, vomiting, and changes in the way things taste and smell. In some cases, the individual experiences symptoms that show the immune system is fighting off the HBV intruder, such as muscle and joint aches, too much protein in the urine, or a rash.

Acute hepatitis B often goes undetected, but that also depends on the age of the person at the time of infection. Its incubation period can be as long as five to six months, and symptoms are vague. If HBV is suspected, the doctor will perform LFTs (liver function tests) and will often find that levels of transaminases (AST and ALT) are elevated. Those levels usually decrease during the course of the disease. If the doctor finds that the AST and ALT are still elevated after six months, it is likely that the illness has progressed from acute to chronic hepatitis B. The best blood tests used to determine whether a person has chronic hepatitis B are persistent hepatitis B sAg or "surface antigen" and the hepatitis B DNA or "viral load." In more than 95 percent of adult acute HBV cases in the United States, the immune system will have conquered the disease and the virus will be gone. Reassurance will come when the above tests return negative results.

In about 1 percent of acute HBV cases – often those acute HBV patients who already have some form of underlying liver disease – the disease may progress to fulminant hepatitis B, a rare but severe occurrence characterized by jaundice, sudden liver failure, coagulopathy (inability to clot blood), and progressive encephalopathy or coma. An immediate liver transplant is needed in order for these patients to survive.

CHRONIC HEPATITIS B

When the HBV continues for more than six months, it is termed chronic hepatitis B. This has the potential to be a more serious form of HBV, because patients whose hepatitis B is chronic can suffer liver damage, cirrhosis, and even liver cancer.

Fortunately, progression from acute to chronic HBV occurs only in about 5 percent of acute adult HBV patients. Researchers aren't sure why some acute HBV patients are able to expel the virus from their bodies, while others – those whose HBV became chronic – are not, but it appears that the immune system does a better job of eliminating HBV in adults than in children. The assumption is that the immune systems of children simply have not matured enough to perform this substantial task, and the numbers affirm it: Infants have only a 5 percent to 10 percent chance of expelling the hepatitis B virus, while children will eliminate it 25 percent to 35 percent of the time, and about 95 percent of adults with acute HBV experience complete spontaneous cures before the virus has a chance to become chronic.

As with acute HBV, the symptoms of chronic HBV are vague: fatigue, weakness, and immune-related disorders such as vasculitis (inflamed blood vessels, hypertension, joint aches, fever, or even kidney failure). Many of these symptoms are referred to as the extrahepatic (meaning "outside the liver") manifestations of chronic hepatitis B.

Usually, chronic hepatitis B is discovered during a routine physical exam or a test for another problem (if, for example, the blood work shows elevated LFTs or the person tried to donate blood and was rejected).

For relatively few people, chronic HBV will progress to cirrhosis before they notice serious symptoms, such as ascites (accumulated fluid in the abdomen), encephalopathy, or liver cancer (hepatocellular carcinoma, or HCC).

Of even greater concern is the fact that in the case of individuals with chronic hepatitis B, hepatocellular carcinoma can develop in the liver even if it is working normally without evidence of cirrhosis.

A minority of patients with chronic hepatitis B develop extrahepatic manifestations of chronic hepatitis B. These extrahepatic symptoms indicate immune-related conditions such as vasculitis (inflammation of the blood vessels) and usually are identified when the person visits the doctor for those ailments, rather than for a liver condition.

Extrahepatic Manifestations of Chronic Hepatitis B	
Serum Sickness-like Syndrome	Fever, skin rashes, and joint pains
Polyarteritis Nodosa	Multiple joint pains and tender skin nodules
Membranous Nephropathy	Kidney disease with protein spilling into the urine

Chronic HBV is diagnosed with a battery of hepatitis B lab tests, actually a series of nearly a dozen different blood tests, which will show whether the person is infectious and confirm that the disease is chronic, among other findings. Those findings usually are supported with results of imaging studies and a liver biopsy.

Patients diagnosed with HBV will often hear the phrase "HBV genotype," which refers to the genetic nature or category of a patient's HBV. There are seven different hepatitis B genotypes, labeled genotype A through G, and each can be identified with a blood test. In the

United States and Europe, genotypes A and D are seen most often, while other genotypes are more prevalent in other parts of the world. The significance of HBV genotypes isn't entirely clear, though researchers are evaluating certain HBV genotypes in terms of the severity of the patient's liver disease and response to treatment.

HEPATITIS B TERMINOLOGY

Chronic hepatitis B is further categorized as (a) inactive hepatitis B surface antigen (HBsAg) carrier state; (b) chronic hepatitis B, either HBeAg positive or HBeAg negative; and (c) resolved chronic hepatitis B.

Patients in the first group, the inactive HBsAg carrier state, typically display no symptoms. They feel fine, their AST and ALT levels are normal, and their livers show no significant damage. Doctors advise them to be tested at least once a year and sometimes more frequently. Their viral load (HBV-DNA level) is usually low.

Chronic HBV patients, the second group, carry HBV DNA, usually at a higher level, meaning that whether they test positive or negative for HBeAg, they are contagious, and their AST/ALT levels remain elevated. HBeAg-positive patients have a small chance (up to 15 percent) of seeing a spontaneous remission.

Those in the third group, individuals diagnosed with resolved chronic HBV, can feel most optimistic about their futures. In patients who resolve, liver enzymes return to normal levels and the risk of developing cirrhosis or liver cancer decreases dramatically. However, if their immune systems ever become deeply suppressed, as happens following chemotherapy or an organ transplant, their chronic hepatitis B can reemerge.

Overall, the long-term prognosis for chronic HBV patients is hopeful: Only about 20 percent develop cirrhosis in the five years following their diagnosis. These rates are variable and depend on where the virus was acquired. Those whose HBV is detected in the early stages seem to fare better, as do those who abstain from alcohol and those who have not also contracted hepatitis C or D.

HEPATITIS D

Hepatitis D (delta hepatitis) is an infection of the liver that exists only in patients with HBV. While it is a rare form of hepatitis, HDV also has a wide variation in presentation. The worst presentation is thought to occur in IV-drug abusers, who may develop severe or fulminant hepatitis.

People with HDV may be infected either through co-infection, meaning that they contracted both HBV and HDV simultaneously, or through superinfection, meaning that they had chronic hepatitis B first and then acquired hepatitis D by continued high-risk behaviors. Almost all HDV patients who acquire the virus at the same time (co-infection) are able to expel both viruses from their bodies, while the opposite is true of those superinfected; up to 95 percent of super-infected HDV patients develop chronic HDV.

TREATING CHRONIC HEPATITIS B AND D

Since in the United States relatively few adult patients with acute hepatitis B develop the chronic form of this hepatitis, generally they are not treated with medications. When HBV patients drink fluids and get plenty of rest, their illness usually resolves on its own.

If the acute hepatitis B has developed into chronic HBV, however, treatment is often prescribed. The majority of patients are treated with daily oral antiviral medications. Others are treated with interferon or sometimes with a long-acting form known as pegylated interferon.

Hepatitis B Treatment with Interferon or Pegylated Interferon

The current recommendation for treatment with pegylated interferon for chronic hepatitis B is 48 weeks of therapy. Unlike the approach in treating chronic hepatitis C, in this case no ribavirin is given. The response rates to treatment vary depending on a number of factors. One of the biggest differences involves whether a person is hepatitis BeAg positive or negative. The side effects of pegylated interferon monotherapy are generally well tolerated, especially in the absence of

HOW PEGYLATED INTERFERON WORKS

The body's natural defenses involve interferon, and many of the symptoms of acute hepatitis are due to the body's natural production of interferon. However, when it is used in regard to treatment with medication, the term "interferon" is a generic term that is used loosely to refer to pegylated interferon 2a or 2b (brand names Pegasys, Peg-Intron). They are different from a standard interferon that was initially researched and used to treat both hepatitis HCV and HBV. It was given three times per week. The short-acting original form of interferon is rarely used to treat HCV or HBV these days. Pegylated interferons were created to stay in the body longer and be "long-acting." They need to be taken only once a week. This long-acting form was created by adding a peg (polyethylene glycol) molecule to standard interferon. This peg delays the drug's excretion by the kidneys.

ribavirin. Studies have shown that the response to interferon therapy (given as subcutaneous injections) is more durable (longer-lasting) than the response achieved with oral antivirals (pills). The durability of the response is one reason some people elect to treat hepatitis B with interferon as opposed to oral medications.

About 40 percent to 60 percent of patients respond favorably, i.e., during therapy the HBV DNA can no longer be found, transaminase levels normalize, and any scarring or inflammation of the liver shows improvement. Many of these patients even "seroconvert" from hepatitis Be antigen (HBeAg) to hepatitis Be antibody (HBeAb). This is felt to be a significantly favorable factor and can improve long-term outcomes.

In some patients, though, interferon therapy can actually cause a transient flare of hepatitis B. This occurs as the body is attempting to rid itself of the virus. If the liver already has extensive damage or is cirrhotic, this flare cannot be tolerated by the ailing liver. The liver will then stop working properly and the person may need an urgent liver transplant. Such individuals are more safely treated with an oral antiviral medicine at the outset.

Hepatitis B Treatment with Oral Antivirals

An alternative to interferon is one of the oral antiviral drugs now available. **Lamivudine** was the first drug in this class and was originally used in treating HIV/AIDS patients. Lamivudine (brand name Epivir-HBV) is a pill with very few side effects and is much more tolerable than interferon. Lamivudine does have two major drawbacks, however. Nearly half of all patients treated with lamivudine will relapse after they stop taking the drug. Even worse, in nearly one-third of patients taking lamivudine, a new strain of HBV evolves and is resistant to lamivudine after the first year. (Lamivudine-resistant strains of HBV are known scientifically as the so-called "YMDD mutations.") The percentage of viral resistance increases the longer the duration of treatment. Viral resistance increases to 60 percent to 70 percent after five years of treatment.

Another drug found effective in treating chronic HBV is **adefovir** (brand name Hepsera), approved by the FDA in 2002. Unlike lamivudine, adefovir does not result in YMDD mutations, but most patients, unfortunately, experience a relapse of their HBV after they stop taking adefovir. Resistance rates for adefovir are somewhat different, depending on the hepatitis Be antigen (HBeAg) status. The estimated cumulative rates of resistance are 0 percent at one year, 3 percent at two years, 11 percent at three years, 18 percent at four years, and 29 percent at five years.

Entecavir (brand name Baraclude) and **telbivudine** (brand name Tyzeka) are two more recent antiviral medications that have been approved to treat chronic hepatitis B in the United States. These newer drugs have been shown to develop resistance at much lower rates than is the case with lamivudine.

Eventually, however, some users of any antiviral drug will develop viral resistance, albeit at different rates. One of the advantages to choosing a newer agent is the lower likelihood of developing a resistance. These newer drugs also have variable degrees of potency and onset of action. The clinician choosing the medication will keep this in mind when selecting the most appropriate therapy. In addition,

COMBINING HEPATITIS B THERAPIES

It seems intuitive that a combination of pegylated interferon with one of the oral antiviral drugs would be more effective than just one therapy in treating chronic hepatitis B. Unfortunately, a number of large, well-designed studies have failed to demonstrate a clear superiority when interferon was combined with oral antiviral medication.

In an alternative approach, different oral antiviral medications are being combined more frequently in an attempt to combat viral resistance.

there can be cross-resistance between certain antivirals, so selection should be performed by a professional well versed in this disease.

In spite of the risks, the vast majority of chronic HBV patients do achieve better health with these drug treatments. Their life expectancy is improved, and their chances of severe complications such as liver cancer or liver failure are greatly diminished. Everyone with chronic HBV should be evaluated, therefore, for these antiviral therapies.

HEPATITIS C – THE "SILENT VIRUS"

It is difficult to imagine having a disease as serious as hepatitis C without knowing you have it, but that's precisely the situation with as many as 60 percent of those infected with the virus. That figure represents a vast number of people – 170 million to 200 million individuals worldwide are estimated to have hepatitis C. In the United States, nearly 15,000 people die every year from complications of HCV, and the U.S. Centers for Disease Control expects that figure to double or possibly even triple over the next 20 years.

Most people think of HCV as being transmitted through the blood during transfusion or intravenous (needle-injection) drug use. But it is possible that it also may be transmitted through intranasal drug use, as in the snorting of cocaine, when tiny blood vessels in the nose burst and the virus gets into the bloodstream. Health-care workers are at risk from a needle "stick," and some cases have been traced to skin penetrations from tattoos or body piercing. While most reputable tattoo parlors are safe, universal precautions are now the standard of care and are observed in the better establishments.

Sexual contact always comes up as a possible mode of transmission. Studies have shown that people with "multiple partners" have a higher risk of acquiring chronic hepatitis C than people who are abstinent or involved in a long-term monogamous relationship. Even so, where there is household contact with a known carrier, individuals should exercise caution with any products that may be exposed to blood or body tissue. No one should share razors or toothbrushes, as these practices can lead to the spread of HCV.

ACUTE HEPATITIS C

Acute hepatitis C resembles acute hepatitis B, in that it is a virus-caused inflammation of the liver that lasts six months or less. Most acute HCV patients exhibit no symptoms at all and are unaware that they are infected. When symptoms do appear, they resemble the flu or many other virus infections: fatigue, weakness, muscle or joint aches, and occasionally a rash. About one-fourth of acute HCV patients exhibit some jaundice (yellowing of the eyes and sometimes skin), providing the clue that the target of this infection is the liver.

When acute HCV is detected with some certainty, it usually is through blood tests. The transaminase levels, AST and ALT, will be elevated for six to eight weeks, then gradually normalize. But bilirubin levels usually are normal, and cholestatic liver enzymes, AP and GGTP, rise only slightly. These LFTs – liver function tests – are not diagnostic tests for hepatitis C, but they do indicate to the doctor that more specific tests to evaluate for hepatitis C might be necessary. The lab tests can sometimes detect antibodies to the HCV virus. The antibody test is the fastest initial screening test and the most easily obtained. For confirmation of viremia (virus present in

INTIMATE CONTACT AND HEPATITIS C

The CDC states in its literature that for monogamous couples engaging in low-risk sexual practices the rate of transmission of HCV is low enough that condoms are not required, provided that the partner of a carrier is aware of the disease.

There is a low probability that a pregnant woman with HCV will pass the virus to her baby. The likelihood increases if the woman is HIV-positive as well as HCV-positive.

It does not appear, however, that breastfeeding mothers with HCV will transmit the disease, so those mothers should not be discouraged from breastfeeding their babies.

the bloodstream), a test that measures the actual hepatitis C genome (HCV RNA) is performed.

There are several types of tests (known by abbreviations such as PCR, TMA, bDNA) that measure the actual amount of hepatitis C RNA virus in the blood. The HCV RNA test, commonly called a "viral load" test, is more expensive than the antibody test. The viral load is the best test to determine whether the virus is present in the bloodstream. This is important as the body sometimes rids itself of the virus on its own. The doctor will want to test the patient again to confirm whether persistent viremia is present.

Six months later, if the HCV RNA has become nondetectable, then patient and doctor will know that it was indeed acute HCV and that the body was able to eliminate the virus on its own. If the immune system has failed to eliminate the HCV, then the hepatitis will have progressed to the stage of chronic infection and treatment options can be explored.

Unfortunately, most acute hepatitis C infections are not identified early because these patients do not frequently seek medical care. The good news is that once a patient is identified as having acute hepatitis C, the treatment is extremely effective. This will be needed if the body's own defenses do not achieve early eradication of the virus. In a number of small studies, treatments for acute hepatitis C have shown a viral eradication rate of up to or greater than 80 percent.

In extremely rare instances, acute HCV develops into a severe form known as fulminant hepatitis C. In fulminant HCV, liver failure, jaundice, and encephalopathy strike suddenly, and the patient must undergo a liver transplant immediately in order to survive.

CHRONIC HEPATITIS C

HCV is a much more stubborn virus than HBV, and up to 85 percent of acute HCV patients may develop chronic hepatitis C. One reason for the resiliency is that the hepatitis C virus found in any one person is actually made up of many genetic variations of HCV, known as hepatitis C quasispecies. Moreover, when the immune system begins fighting the HCV virus, the virus it encounters is devious and may change its genetic features in subtle ways, thereby evading the body's defenses.

People may be infected with chronic HCV for years and not know it. Only about 25 percent of HCV-infected persons notice any symptoms at all, and those that they do notice are likely to be mild and rather nonspecific, such as weakness, weight loss, some depression, and possibly discomfort in the abdomen. As many people have no troublesome symptoms, the diagnosis of hepatitis C may be made incidentally, for example when a life-insurance physical calls for lab tests, or when a blood donation is taken by the American Red Cross.

Chronic HCV sometimes causes disorders outside the liver. These are called extrahepatic manifestations. Skin diseases, such as vasculitis (inflammation of blood vessels), blisters, and pruritus (extreme itching) are some of these rarer features. Blood-related disorders, such as non-Hodgkin's B-cell lymphoma, may be seen. Thyroid disease, diabetes, corneal ulcers, kidney disorders, and joint pain are other disorders possibly associated with chronic HCV.

When chronic HCV is suspected, the doctor will obtain several tests to determine the best course of treatment of the disease. The first test is hepatitis C viral RNA (HCV RNA), which confirms the presence of the virus in the blood (viremia). Next the doctor can choose from a number of tests that will assess the actual "viral load," or amount of HCV RNA in 1 ml of blood. These quantitative tests include the polymerase chain reaction (PCR), target-mediated amplification (TMA), and branched DNA (bDNA) – three simple blood tests with long, confusing names. Usually these tests are reported in international units per milliliter of blood, or IU/ml.

Another term often associated with HCV is "genotype," referring to the genetic makeup of an individual's specific strain of HCV. Researchers recognize six clear HCV genotypes, and a patient's genotype is identified with a simple blood test. Genotypes are reported as 1 through 6, with subgroups indicated by lowercase letters a, b, c. In rare instances people can be infected by more than one genotype.

While a genotype cannot predict the seriousness or course of a person's HCV, certain genotypes do respond to interferon therapy better than others do. Genotype 1, the most common genotype in the United States, is considered the most difficult to treat. Genotypes 2 and 3 generally are easier to treat than genotype 1, require less medication, and have a shorter course of therapy. Genotype 4, mostly found in Egypt, is treated the way genotype 1 is treated. Genotype 5 which is more common in Africa, and genotype 6, more common in Asia, are also treated the way genotype 1 is treated.

Doctors will usually order an imaging study of the liver to detect a possible mass, ascites, varices, and other abnormalities.

Doctors will usually order an imaging study of the liver to detect a possible mass, ascites, varices, and other abnormalities. The best information about liver inflammation, scarring or fibrosis (cirrhosis) damage, and the possibility of other coexisting liver diseases is obtained through a liver biopsy. (See Chapter 13 for information on liver biopsies.)

VIRAL LOADS AND LIVER DAMAGE

One might think that a higher viral load would cause more damage to a liver than a lower one would cause. This is not true. The value of a viral load is in its ability to let us know how well a person might respond to antiviral therapy (pegylated interferon and ribavirin). People with "low viral loads" usually respond better and can sometimes require less medication. There are different definitions for what constitutes a "low viral load," but generally it is considered to be < 600,000 IU/mL to < 800,000 IU/mL.

AFTER A DIAGNOSIS OF CHRONIC HCV

It is both good news and bad news: Chronic hepatitis C can take up to 20, 30, even 50 years before any significant liver damage is evident. The patient might live normally, with no symptoms, for decades without suspecting the presence of a potentially serious disease. It is possible to live out one's entire adult life without ever discovering the "silent virus." Unfortunately, that also means that chronic HCV can progress to a more serious stage before it is detected.

Overall, most chronic HCV patients do not develop cirrhosis until 20 to 30 years after they contract the disease. Even then, they can lead normal, active lives unless a serious complication such as variceal bleeding, ascites, or encephalopathy has developed.

Personal characteristics seem to affect the course of the disease. Women generally develop cirrhosis less commonly than men, and those who contract HCV at a younger age (under 40) also are less likely to see advanced scarring.

Lifestyle is a very important factor in the prognosis of chronic HCV patients. Alcohol can be toxic to the liver and in fact can accelerate the progression of liver damage in cases of chronic HCV. So while there have been conflicting reports and studies regarding a "safe amount of alcohol" in patients with chronic hepatitis C, it is prudent to avoid alcohol altogether if one has a chronic progressive liver disease.

Those who smoke cigarettes may display more scarring and inflammation in their biopsies and tend to develop liver cancer slightly faster than nonsmokers.

Obesity, which is reaching epidemic proportions in the industrialized world, is also an issue that should be addressed. Studies have indicated an increased incidence of cirrhosis and liver cancer in obese patients. Education and other methods of weight control are recommended.

Chronic HCV also occurs in persons who are HIV-positive. For these patients, there is an increased risk of acquiring both diseases as they are both blood-borne illnesses. Recently, there has been an increased incidence of HIV/HCV co-infected patients developing significant liver disease. Currently available highly active antiretroviral therapy, or HAART, has been effective in prolonging the lives of patients living with HIV. Now that HIV/HCV co-infected patients are living longer and not dying from the complications of AIDS, many are progressing to end-stage liver disease. This observation has led to several large international trials that have demonstrated the effectiveness of pegylated interferon and ribavirin in the treatment of co-infected patients. Historically, this group of HIV/HCV co-infected patients has been undertreated for chronic hepatitis C. In light of current literature and the demonstrated safety and effectiveness of modern therapy, there is no reason that co-infected patients should not be evaluated for hepatitis C treatment.

Another issue that can make the treatment of HCV more difficult is the concept of an overlap of liver diseases. Overlap simply means that there are two distinct processes or diseases occurring in the liver at the same time. In some cases this can cause significant issues in regard to medication selection. We sometimes see an overlap between chronic HCV and other liver diseases, such as autoimmune hepatitis (AIH), nonalcoholic fatty liver disease (NAFLD), and hemochromatosis (iron overload). While not all of these overlaps suggest a more serious progression of liver damage for chronic HCV per se, they often do present tricky situations in the treatment of two (or more) diseases.

Common Terms in Chronic Hepatitis C Therapy	
Genotype	Essentially the strain of hepatitis. There are six major genotypes with subtypes denoted by lowercase letters (e.g., genotype 1b). Genotype 1 is more difficult to treat than genotypes 2 or 3 and has a lower response rate.
Viral Load	The amount of virus in 1 milliliter of blood, reported as international units (IU) per milliliter (ml). A high viral load is harder to treat than a low viral load.
Rapid Virologic Response (RVR)	Hepatitis C virus (HCV RNA) is nondetectable after four weeks of pegylated interferon and ribavirin therapy.
Early Virologic Response (EVR)	Hepatitis C virus (HCV RNA) reduction is greater than 2 logs (more than a hundredfold) from baseline after 12 weeks of pegylated interferon and ribavirin therapy.
End-of-Treatment Response (ETR)	Hepatitis C virus (HCV RNA) is nondetectable after the completion of pegylated interferon and ribavirin therapy.
Sustained Viral Response (SVR)	Hepatitis C virus (HCV RNA) is nondetectable six months or more after the completion of therapy with pegylated interferon and ribavirin therapy. Essentially a cure for about 99% of patients.

TREATMENT OF HCV

For chronic HCV, the most effective treatment is antiviral therapy – that is, medication that targets a virus. Interferon, a widely known antiviral discussed earlier in this chapter, is the treatment of choice for chronic HCV.

Pegylated Interferon and Ribavirin Therapy

The combination of pegylated interferon 2a or 2b (brand names Pegasys, Peg-Intron) and ribavirin is currently the "standard of care" for treating patients with chronic hepatitis C. It should be mentioned that there is in current use one type of *daily* interferon known as consensus interferon (brand name Infergen). It is taken seven days a week in combination with ribavirin. This drug is generally reserved for patients who fail pegylated interferon and ribavirin.

While pegylated interferon in combination with ribavirin is the most effective treatment for chronic hepatitis C, the side effects can be substantial. Flulike symptoms (fever, chills, muscle and joint pain, fatigue) are common, and doctors often prescribe medications to combat these symptoms if they become debilitating. It is also important for patients to maintain their activity levels – even though they may feel too weak to move much – to build a little muscle and be able to muster the energy to get through the day. Adequate fluid intake is also essential. This is a simple and often overlooked strategy. Many patients report that substantially increasing their daily fluid intake is the most effective method in combating the flulike side effects that plague pegylated interferon-based therapy.

Depression, insomnia, irritability, and even confusion are experienced by more than half of all patients undergoing interferon therapy. For some, antidepressant medications might be appropriate. This depression is considered to be somewhat different from classic major depression. The depression that is caused by taking interferon generally responds more briskly to typical antidepressants such as citalopram (brand name Celexa) or sertraline (brand name Zoloft).

Thyroid disorders also occur in some patients during interferon therapy, both underfunctioning thyroid (hypothyroidism) and overfunctioning thyroid (hyperthyroidism). Symptoms of hypothyroidism – hair loss, sensations of coldness, weight gain, fatigue, dry skin – are easily treated with medicine, as is hyperthyroidism (anxiety, weight loss, shortness of breath). Chronic hepatitis C patients who are taking pegylated interferon and ribavirin therapy should be encouraged to

Common Side Effects of Pegylated Interferon and Ribavirin Therapy	
SIDE EFFECT	TREATMENT
Fatigue	Rest, increase fluid intake
Depression	Maintain exercise, use medication if needed
Irritability	Employ coping strategies, use medications if needed
Anemia	Reduce ribavirin, use growth factors such as erythropoietin (Procrit, Epogen, Aranesp)
Neutropenia	Reduce interferon dose, use growth factors such as filgrastim (Neupogen)
Thinning hair	Use gentle soaps, avoid permanents or hair coloring
Thyroid problems	Lab tests will determine type; use medications if needed
Dry skin	Use moisturizing lotions liberally, avoid harsh chemicals or excessive sunlight

have their thyroid function tested about every three months; thyroid disorders can be diagnosed with simple blood tests.

Other side effects that don't seem to follow any regular pattern include headaches, vision problems or dry eyes, weight changes, brittle nails, insomnia, changes in blood levels, a burning sensation in the mouth (known as stomatitis), decreased sex drive, and menstrual irregularities. All of these symptoms are to some degree manageable. In some patients the side effects can be severe, and supportive medications are able only to "take the edge off." Although treatment may be difficult, centers that regularly treat chronic hepatitis C are well versed in managing the side effects. These centers will also maintain the proper dose of medication and ensure that patients have the best possible chance to permanently rid their bodies of the virus.

Because of chronic HCV's complicated makeup – remember the genotypes? – pegylated interferon therapy must be customized. Therapy duration is dictated by the genotype. Pegylated interferon is always used, if possible, in combination with ribavirin. The only time ribavirin is not used is when there is a medical contraindication, such as chronic renal (kidney) failure requiring dialysis, or a severe allergy to ribavirin. How well the patient is responding to antiviral treatment is determined by two simple lab tests. The first is the alanine transaminase (ALT) test. When the ALT decreases and returns to a normal level, it is referred to as a biochemical response. This does not always occur, but is a considered good sign. The most important test in determining treatment success is the HCV RNA, or viral load test. The decline in the viral load is the most crucial aspect of therapy. One must first have a baseline or pre-treatment viral load to measure against the subsequent or on-treatment viral loads.

Treatment of Genotypes 1, 4, 5, and 6

The first viral load to be measured after treatment commences comes after four weeks of therapy (one month). If the viral load is nondetectable at one month, this is referred to as a rapid virologic response

GROWTH FACTORS

"Growth factors" are medicines that are used to increase the bone marrow's production of red blood cells (RBC's) or white blood cells (WBC's) during the treatment of chronic hepatitis C. These drugs attempt to combat the anemia and neutropenia (low white blood cell count) that are frequently caused by pegylated interferon and ribavirin therapy. Examples include erythropoietin and filgrastim (brand names shown in the box on page 30). Sometimes there is difficulty in obtaining these growth factors, which are approved by the FDA, but not specifically for the treatment of anemia or neutropenia that results from the use of pegylated interferon and ribavirin.

or RVR. People who achieve an RVR are called "super responders." They have an excellent chance of eradicating the virus after they complete their treatment. A small subset of patients with a low viral load who achieve an RVR (HCV RNA negativity after four weeks of treatment) can sometimes be given a choice to stop treatment early. The determination to stop treatment early is usually made on a case-by-case basis and the patient should be presented with the pros and cons of this approach.

The next step is to measure the viral load after 12 weeks (three months) of therapy. The result of this viral load test is referred to by different names, depending on the results. When the virus is nondetectable after three months of therapy, it is referred to as a complete early virologic response (cEVR). If the viral load has declined by two logs but is still detectable, it is referred to as a partial early virologic response (pEVR).

People who achieve a partial or complete early virologic response are able to continue therapy. Those who do not achieve a two-log reduction after 12 weeks are considered nonresponders (NR). Unfortunately, it is known that nonresponders have less than a 3 percent chance of obtaining a sustained viral response (SVR) even if they complete the full course of therapy. Therefore, therapy is stopped for nonresponders (NR) after three months if they do not obtain a two-log reduction.

For patients who remain on therapy, the next viral load is measured after six months (24 weeks) of therapy. This viral load must be nondetectable or negative, or treatment is usually stopped. If the viral load is measurable to any degree after six months, treatment is generally discontinued as these patients will almost never achieve treatment success even if they complete the full 48 weeks of therapy.

After completion of 48 weeks of pegylated interferon and ribavirin another viral load is obtained. This viral load is referred to as the end-of-treatment response (ETR). This viral load marks the end of therapy and the waiting game begins. For treatment to be considered a success, the viral load must remain negative for at least six months after the end of therapy. Unfortunately some patients will test positive during this six-month period; they are referred to as relapsers. Relapsers should follow up and discuss their situation with a hepatologist.

If a patient completes therapy, waits six months, and remains virologically negative, this is regarded as a sustained virologic response (SVR) and the treatment is considered a success. For patients who achieve an SVR, a relapse is highly unlikely. This is essentially the same as a cure for 97 percent to 99 percent of patients.

A word of caution regarding lab tests: If a person achieves a sustained virology response (SVR), the virus will remain nondetectable. However, the antibody test does not change and may remain positive for life. The antibody is the "footprint" of previous infection. It informs us only that the patient was exposed to the virus; it does not indicate active infection. Many times this lab test is obtained in error and can cause confusion and fear in patients. If you have obtained a sustained viral response (SVR) and are told you have the virus again, please call your hepatologist to confirm this finding.

Treatment of Genotypes 2 and 3

Genotypes 2 and 3 require only six months (24 weeks) of therapy with lower doses of ribavirin. Viral loads are checked after one month (4 weeks), three months (12 weeks) and six months (24 weeks). The same rules apply in determining whether the patient achieves a sustained viral response (SVR). One must wait for six months after therapy has ended and must have a negative or nondetectable viral load.

INTERCHANGEABLE TERMS

Viral loads are reported from the lab as positive (with a numerical value) or nondetectable. Many clinicians tell their patients that the test result is negative. For the purposes of this book the terms can be used interchangeably.

NONRESPONDERS HAVE OPTIONS

Nonresponders should not give up hope. People who are nonresponders or relapsers still have options. The first option is to consider asking for a referral to an academic or research institution. The medical records of the previous treatment(s) should be obtained and reviewed to make certain that the medications were given in the proper doses and for the proper duration. One option is to consider a daily interferon treatment with a drug called consensus interferon (brand name Infergen) in combination with ribavirin.

Another alternative is to become enrolled in a clinical trial. All new and potentially more effective medications have to be researched. Large medical centers frequently have a number of ongoing clinical trials of newer treatments that are not as yet approved by the FDA. These trials are usually conducted under FDA and/or NIH supervision.

The third option is watchful waiting. Healthful living is important and is strongly encouraged. If one does not already have cirrhosis, a repeat biopsy may be obtained in three to five years to assess progression or lack of progression of disease. ◆

Chapter 3

Autoimmune Hepatitis

Marti knew that something was wrong. She felt tired all the time, and her joints ached every day. The 20-year-old college senior, a graphic design major, thought she might even be able to diagnose the cause of her sluggishness herself.

Although Marti's weight was in the "average" range, her mother had been obese for as long as Marti could remember. Several years earlier, her mom had been diagnosed with Hashimoto's thyroiditis: underactive thyroid, the primary symptom of which was fatigue. Another frequent symptom was soreness in the joints. Marti knew that thyroiditis, an autoimmune disorder, was influenced by genetics. Had she simply "inherited" her mother's thyroid disease?

When blood tests failed to reveal thyroiditis, Marti's doctor began testing for other diseases that were likely to display the same symptoms. Through a process of elimination, Marti eventually was diagnosed with autoimmune hepatitis, a disease in which the patient's own immune system begins attacking the liver. Because she consulted her doctor early and was able to undergo aggressive treatment, her prospects for a liver-healthy future appear to be good.

THE MANY DISGUISES OF HEPATITIS

Some of the most troubling illnesses are those whose symptoms are common. What busy person would visit a doctor for fatigue? Or for joint pains, spider veins, easy bruising, or itchy skin? Yet these all can be symptoms of autoimmune hepatitis (AIH), a condition that can be controlled for years if detected early and treated appropriately. If the symptoms are allowed to continue, though, the disease will progress and the outcome might not be so positive.

Like all autoimmune diseases, autoimmune hepatitis is a disease in which the patient's immune system rebels and instead of being protective goes on the attack – in this case, attacking the liver. It manifests as a progressive inflammation and usually strikes women (70 percent of the time). For years it was thought to be a form of lupus, another autoimmune disease. In fact, it was called "lupoid hepatitis" in the earliest descriptions. No one knows the exact cause, or why it is usually women who contract this disease. Researchers now suspect that a genetic predisposition might be assisted by some event that triggers the disease, such as an infection or the use of some medications.

Most commonly, doctors will find that the patient or perhaps a close family member already suffers from an autoimmune disease, such as rheumatoid arthritis, lupus, or thyroid disease. The symptoms of AIH – including deep fatigue, aching joints, and dry, itchy skin – often mirror the symptoms of those other disorders. Other signs of AIH might be abdominal discomfort, spider angiomas (enlarged blood vessels) on the face and upper body, vomiting, dark urine, jaundice, and Sjögren's syndrome (a disorder characterized by dry eyes and mouth). The disease often strikes young women in their teen or early adult years.

DIAGNOSING AIH

Pinpointing AIH is often a process of elimination requiring a battery of tests, as no single test has yet been devised to diagnose AIH specifically. When a series of diagnostic procedures is performed, other liver diseases can be eliminated and AIH can be confirmed.

Doctors will begin with liver function tests (LFTs), producing an alphabet soup of results: The transaminase levels (AST and ALT) will be tested, and if AIH is present, will be shown to be elevated. GGTP (gamma-glutamyl transpeptidase) and alkaline phosphatase (AP) tests will be made, and while the AP may be normal, frequently it is elevated.

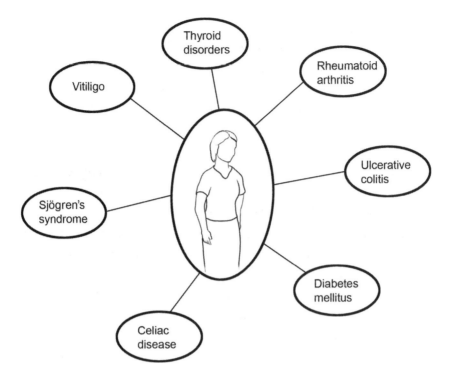

Hepatitis unmasked: *People with autoimmune hepatitis often have one or more of the autoimmune conditions indicated above. Only extensive testing can establish a reliable diagnosis.*

Autoimmune blood tests will be scheduled to check for a high gamma globulin or immunoglobulin G (IgG) level. AIH usually will produce gamma globulin or IgG levels that are well above the normal range. These autoimmune blood tests also measure autoantibodies – antinuclear antibodies (ANA), smooth muscle antibodies (SMA), and the liver-kidney-microsomal antibody (anti-LKM) – another alphabet soup. While it is certainly not necessary for the patient to memorize the chemistry of liver testing, it can be immensely reassuring to understand the technical background of the tests and to know the roles that these substances play.

Patients should understand that autoantibodies do not cause AIH, but that people with AIH produce autoantibodies. The most common autoantibodies are ANA and SMA, which are found in most AIH patients. However, both ANA and SMA occur in other liver diseases, typically in a lower concentration, and to a lesser degree in diseases of other organs, such as lupus or rheumatoid arthritis – which is why it is necessary to test first for ANA and SMA, and then to let those results guide further testing.

Genetic markers may be important when a diagnosis of AIH is considered, because there is an apparent genetic connection between AIH and the human leukocyte antigens (HLAs) found on chromosome number 6.

HLAs are special substances determined by genes on our chromosomes that can help us predict a person's tendency to contract different diseases. Two HLAs (DR3 and DR4) found on chromosome 6 are related to AIH. Not every medical laboratory is equipped to test for these HLAs, but when other factors in an AIH diagnosis are uncertain, testing for HLAs can help lead to an accurate diagnosis.

When all other testing points to AIH, a liver biopsy will confirm the diagnosis and accurately show the amount of damage to the liver that the disease has caused. (Liver biopsy is discussed at length in Chapter 14.) On the basis of this information, the physician team will devise a treatment plan.

OVERLAPPING DIAGNOSES

In many instances, a patient will show symptoms of AIH along with symptoms of other autoimmune diseases affecting the liver. When this "overlap syndrome" occurs, treatment decisions are not so clearcut. Usually, doctors opt to treat the disease showing the strongest features. When test results show that two autoimmune liver diseases coexist in more or less equal intensity, they will combine treatment therapies to address both diseases.

Three autoimmune liver diseases commonly overlap with AIH: primary biliary cirrhosis (PBC), primary sclerosing cholangitis (PSC), and autoimmune cholangitis, while viral hepatitis, particularly hepatitis B and C (HBV and HCV), may also show features similar to AIH.

The blood of AIH patients suspected of having PBC (about 10 percent of AIH patients) contains the antimitochondrial antibody (AMA), which is present almost invariably in PBC. A small proportion of AIH patients, about 6 percent, also show symptoms of PSC, marked by narrowing and dilation in both the intrahepatic and extra-hepatic bile ducts. PSC occurs most often in men, while AIH is most often found in women, so that AIH patients – especially men, and especially those suffering from ulcerative colitis, which is linked to PSC – should be tested for PSC. Most patients with AIH and PSC overlap syndrome are the youngest AIH patients, but PSC also can develop in older AIH patients who have been able to control their illness for years. If the AIH treatment seems to be no longer effective, testing for PSC should be considered.

Another autoimmune disease that inflames the liver (as well as injuring the bile ducts and showing ANA or SMA) is autoimmune cholangitis (autoimmune cholangiopathy), sometimes treated with steroids. AIH also frequently overlaps with chronic HBV and HCV. Patients displaying this syndrome may require careful assessment of both conditions. A liver biopsy is used to determine whether they need to be treated with antivirals or with medications to treat the autoimmune process. In this situation, patients are treated according to the progression of their HBV or HCV, including with a program of interferon when appropriate.

TREATING AIH

Like most autoimmune diseases, AIH is a chronic condition, but the good news is that once diagnosed, it usually can be controlled with a low-maintenance dose of prednisone, a corticosteroid, or synthetic steroid. Another common prescription for AIH is azathioprine (Imuran). Both drugs aim to suppress the overactive immune system, thus keeping AIH under control.

Some patients may need to take prednisone for the rest of their lives, starting with a higher initial dose and tapering off once AIH is in remission, usually less than two years after the diagnosis. For most, though, it is best to switch to azathioprine when possible because of prednisone's side effects, including weight gain, osteoporosis, thinning hair and skin, diabetes, high blood pressure, cataracts, glaucoma, anxiety, and confusion. More than 40 percent of patients taking the drug long-term will experience at least one of those side effects. Azathioprine, too, can bring its own side effects, including nausea, loss of appetite, pancreatitis, allergic reaction, and a lower white blood cell count.

In spite of those unpleasant possibilities, some combination of the two drugs effectively controls AIH about 75 percent of the time. Many patients feel stronger and better after only two weeks of drug treatment. When the drugs succeed, a liver biopsy will show decreased inflammation and scarring.

For the remaining patients, who don't respond well to drug therapy for AIH, other immunosuppressive drugs (including mycophenolate mofetil, cyclosporine, and tacrolimus) have sometimes been effective. If those substances also fail and the liver deteriorates, the best option may be a liver transplant.

A POSITIVE PROGNOSIS

AIH patients should plan on long-term therapy, which will probably call for a lifetime commitment. Of those who do stop treatment, about 50 percent relapse within six months after discontinuing their medication. Those who don't relapse have an 80 percent chance of remaining AIH-free, but the others usually go back to a low dosage of prednisone, azathioprine, or both.

A minority of patients on drug therapy (up to 20 percent) never do respond positively to the treatment. Drugs aren't always recommended for those with mild AIH, which is defined as having near-normal transaminases and minimal inflammation on biopsy. Nor are drugs always recommended for patients diagnosed with cirrhosis but without inflammation in the liver, or for patients with mild hepatitis. Ironically, the more severe the symptoms, the greater the expected benefit from drug therapy for AIH.

Postmenopausal women often are cautioned against taking prednisone because of the risk of developing osteoporosis. Also, severe AIH can cause a woman to stop menstruating, so female patients of child-bearing age who do *not* undergo drug therapy might not be able to become pregnant. The menstrual cycles usually normalize, however, with corticosteroids and azathioprine, and the patient once again becomes able to conceive.

AIH is a disease in which so many factors influence each other that it is difficult to make generalizations about a long-term prognosis. Studies have shown, though, that patients who do not seek treatment for severe AIH have only a 30 percent chance of surviving beyond five years. Those who undergo drug therapy have an 11 percent risk of seeing their AIH progress to cirrhosis during the first three years of treatment. Once the three-year milestone has passed, the risk shrinks dramatically, to 1 percent each year.

RELATIONSHIPS AND DISGUISES

Like all autoimmune diseases, AIH is associated with many other autoimmune disorders. Any patient with AIH has a 50 percent chance of also contracting another autoimmune disease. The list is long:

- Thyroid disorders, specifically hyperthyroidism (overactive thyroid) and hypothyroidism (underactive thyroid)
- Rheumatoid arthritis
- Ulcerative colitis (inflammation of the large intestine, or colon)
- Diabetes mellitus
- Blood disorders, including anemia and a low platelet count
- Celiac sprue, or intolerance to wheat gluten
- Myasthenia gravis, a neuromuscular disease
- Sjögren's syndrome, a disease marked by dry eyes and mouth
- Vitiligo, a disorder that creates discolored skin patches

It also should be noted that the same symptoms present in patients with AIH are also commonly found in a host of other illnesses and conditions. If you are experiencing any of these symptoms, it is important to consult a doctor and discuss other diagnostic possibilities. ◆

Chapter 4

Nonalcoholic Fatty Liver Disease

As Jessie leaned against her kitchen counter, reaching for her blender, she felt again a vague discomfort in the upper right area of her stomach. It wasn't a sharp pain; it was more of a tender, full feeling in her upper abdomen. Jessie didn't have much of a medical background, but she knew that the only important organ in that region was her liver. The soreness scared her.

Jessie didn't want to see a doctor for this problem. At 53 and with no health insurance, she feared that if her doctor uncovered a serious problem requiring a hospital stay, she'd lose her house. Self-employed florists don't make the kind of money that would cover lengthy treatments. So she put the discomfort out of her mind until she could figure out what to do.

In the meantime, Jessie began taking long walks around her neighborhood. Always a hefty woman, she had noticed increasing soreness in her knees and a little too much sag in her neck. Her weight aged her, both in her appearance and the way she felt, so she started eating less fat and more vegetables and whole grains. After a few months, she had dropped 15 pounds – just enough to notice a difference in her knees and the way her clothes fit – and she no longer felt the pain in her abdomen. Jessie forgot that she had ever felt that soreness, and she never did learn that she probably had had nonalcoholic fatty liver disease.

AMERICA'S NEWEST HEALTH CRISIS?

With concern growing over epidemic obesity in America, it's no surprise that nonalcoholic fatty liver disease (NAFLD), most often found in people who are overweight or obese, is the most common liver disease in the United States, with an estimated 10 percent to 40 percent of the general global population affected. Up to 75 percent of obese persons, 50 percent of people with diabetes, and 90 percent of morbidly obese people – those weighing in at more than 200 percent of their ideal body weight – are said to have NAFLD. It is estimated that in the United States more than 30 million adults have NAFLD and nearly 9 million have nonalcoholic steatohepatitis (NASH), far surpassing cases of chronic hepatitis C, which has been diagnosed in 4 million adults in the United States. NAFLD also is found in children: It has been estimated that some 53 percent of obese children have fatty liver disease.

There was a time when it was believed that both fatty liver and cirrhosis were caused by laziness and lack of self-control: "Fatty degeneration of the liver," wrote one C. Murchison in 1885, "is well known to be a common lesion in persons who are large feeders or drink much alcohol and lead indolent lives."

NAFLD develops in two stages. The first, a simple fatty liver, is relatively harmless and reversible, and need not ever lead to cirrhosis or liver cancer. Once it progresses to NASH, however – nonalcoholic steatohepatitis, in which the liver becomes inflamed and then scarred – the disease has reached a more dangerous level and can be the cause of cirrhosis, liver cancer, and liver failure.

NAFLD is found in every demographic group, though its primary targets are women in their middle years who carry too much weight and who also may have high cholesterol and triglyceride levels. Technically, a liver is found to be "fatty" when fat makes up at least 10 percent of the liver. (The point should be made that eating fatty food alone will not produce a fatty liver; many people who eat high-fat diets are not obese and don't have fatty liver.)

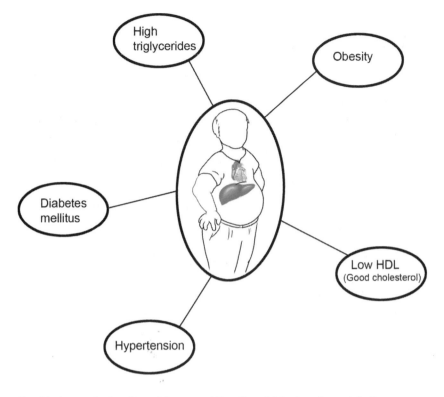

Double jeopardy: *Insulin resistance and the other risk factors for metabolic syndrome significantly increase an individual's chance of developing nonalcoholic fatty liver disease (NAFLD).*

Picture the French delicacy *pâté de foie gras* and how it is produced. In 1842 the German chemist Justus von Liebig underlined the importance of exercise to human liver health when he likened the development of human fatty liver disease to the fattening of a goose: With its feet tied to prevent it from exercising, the goose is force-fed until its liver is "soft and spongy."

Obesity, though, can contribute to fatty liver because obese people may store fat in every area of their bodies, including the liver. Ironically, fatty liver may also occur in people who lose weight too quickly. The liver may not be able to handle the huge task of breaking down all that fat in the tissues, so it simply accumulates it – a little-known argument for a more measured approach to weight reduction!

WHAT IS BMI?

Body Mass Index (BMI) is a number calculated from a person's weight and height. BMI is a reliable indicator of body fatness for people. BMI does not measure body fat directly, but research has shown that BMI correlates to direct measures of body fat, such as underwater weighing and dual energy x-ray absorptiometry (DXA). BMI can be considered an alternative for direct measures of body fat. Additionally, BMI is an inexpensive and easy-to-perform method of screening for weight categories that may lead to health problems.

HOW IS BMI CALCULATED AND INTERPRETED?

Calculation of BMI

BMI is calculated the same way for adults and children. The calculation is based on the following formulas:

Measurement Units	Formula and Calculation
Kilograms and and meters (or centimeters)	**Formula** – weight (kg) / [height (m)]2 With the metric system, the formula for BMI is weight in kilograms divided by height in meters squared. Since height is commonly measured in centimeters, divide height in centimeters by 100 to obtain height in meters: **e.g.,** Weight = 68 kg, Height = 165 cm (1.65 m) **Calculation** – 68 ÷ (1.65)2 = 24.98
Pounds and inches	**Formula** – weight (lb) / [height (in)]2 x 703 Calculate BMI by dividing weight in pounds (lbs) by height in inches (in) squared and multiplying by a conversion factor of 703: **e.g.,** Weight = 150 lbs, Height = 5'5"(65") **Calculation** – [150 ÷ (65)2] x 703 = 24.96

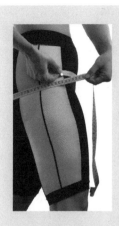

Interpretation of BMI for Adults

For adults 20 years old and older, BMI is interpreted using standard weight status categories that are the same for all ages and for both men and women. For children and teens, on the other hand, the interpretation of BMI is both age- and sex-specific. For more information about interpretation for children and teens, visit the Child and Teen BMI Calculator at www.cdc.gov/nccdphp/dnpa/bmi/.

The standard weight status categories associated with BMI ranges for adults are shown in the following table.

BMI	Weight Status
Below 18.5	Underweight
18.5 – 24.9	Normal
25.0 – 29.9	Overweight
30.0 and above	Obese

For example, here are the weight ranges, the corresponding BMI ranges, and the weight status categories for a sample height.

Height	Weight Range	BMI	Weight Status
5' 9"	124 lbs or less	Below 18.5	Underweight
	125 lbs to 168 lbs	18.5 to 24.9	Normal
	169 lbs to 202 lbs	25.0 to 29.9	Overweight
	203 lbs or more	30 or higher	Obese

The above information can be found at the Centers for Disease Control website. For this and more, go to http://www.cdc.gov/nccdphp/dnpa/bmi/.

NAFLD can't be traced to a single cause, though the metabolic syndrome (see below) is the primary risk factor – and that risk increases as body weight climbs. More than 70 percent of NASH patients are obese, which is defined as having a body mass index (BMI) of 30 or higher. (Overweight is defined as having a BMI of 25 to 30.)

To calculate your BMI, divide your weight (in pounds) by your height in inches squared, and multiply that number by 703. If your BMI falls between 20 and 24.9, your weight is in the "normal" range. You're considered overweight if you have a BMI of 25 to 29.9 and obese if your BMI falls between 30 and 39.9. Persons with a BMI over 40 are categorized as "morbidly obese."

INSULIN RESISTANCE

Insulin resistance poses another major risk. Insulin is the substance that keeps our glucose (blood sugar) levels from becoming too elevated by guiding the glucose from our bloodstream into the body's muscle, fat, and liver cells. The cells convert the glucose into energy, but if the glucose isn't metabolized correctly (i.e., if the cells *resist* the insulin and won't allow it to do its job) then we produce less energy and feel fatigued.

People who are insulin resistant can't use insulin efficiently, and glucose builds in the blood – in which case the pancreas produces even more insulin, trying to rid the body of the excess glucose. The end result is an abundance of fatty acids that are converted to fat, which is stored in the liver, creating NAFLD. Almost all people with NAFLD are insulin resistant. It is also believed that even though overweight people are more likely to exhibit insulin resistance than those of normal weight, a sedentary lifestyle and a high-fat, high-sugar diet triggers insulin resistance regardless of body weight or BMI.

This combination of factors and related disorders of metabolism (obesity, insulin resistance, diabetes, hypertriglyceridemia, and hypertension) comprises the group of findings known as the metabolic syndrome. People with the metabolic syndrome generally also have NAFLD, which in some cases will have progressed to NASH.

NAFLD OR NASH?

The acronyms can be confusing. One way to distinguish between NAFLD and NASH is to put them into alphabetical order, in which case NAFLD, or fatty liver disease, comes before NASH, or nonalcoholic steatohepatitis. This is helpful to remember because it reflects the order in which the two diseases work: Fatty liver disease arises first and can progress to nonalcoholic steatohepatitis.

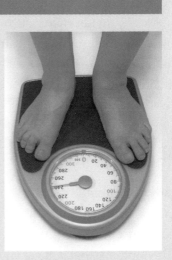

Here are some facts at a glance:

- Simple fatty liver (which is just what the words imply, an accumulation of fat in the liver) is the beginning stage of NAFLD. It is caused by insulin resistance, meaning that the insulin produced in the body is less effective than it should be. The primary factor in the development of insulin resistance is obesity, especially central obesity.

- Simple fatty liver is relatively harmless and often disappears with weight loss.

- The next stage of NAFLD is NASH. When NASH occurs, the liver is still fatty, but it also becomes inflamed (hepatitis) and liver cells can be destroyed. It can progress to scarring of the liver (fibrosis) and development of severe liver diseases, including cirrhosis, which is the last stage of NAFLD.

- The Centers for Disease Control estimates that an astonishing 90 percent of people who are obese or have been diagnosed with type 2 diabetes also have simple fatty liver. About 20 percent of them have NASH, and 10 percent have cirrhosis.

There are other, less common causes of NAFLD. One is "drug-induced steatohepatitis," or more precisely "drug-induced fatty liver," caused by medications such as prednisone (a steroid), tamoxifen (used in treating breast cancer), estrogen (a female hormone), methotrexate (used to treat cancer and autoimmune conditions), amiodarone (used to treat heart conditions), or Arimidex (used to treat breast cancer).

DETECTING NAFLD

Early symptoms of fatty liver disease are vague and nonspecific: fatigue, malaise, the ache in the upper right abdomen that Jessie experienced.

Symptoms that appear in the advanced stages of NASH mimic those of cirrhosis; they range from fluid in the abdominal cavity (ascites), severe itching, swelling (edema) of the legs and feet, and weakness to nausea, easy bruising, yellowing of the skin and eyes (jaundice), dark (cola-colored) urine, and mental confusion.

The ache in the upper-right abdomen is a signal that the liver may be swollen, and that is the point when individuals should see a doctor. The physician may prescribe blood tests to rule out other liver-damaging conditions, including hepatitis B and C. You also may be asked about your consumption of alcohol, to assess whether your drinking may be excessive (defined as three or more drinks a day for men and two or more drinks for women); this also can cause fatty liver and ASH (alcoholic steatohepatitis).

The ache in the upper-right abdomen is a signal that the liver may be swollen, and that is the point when individuals should see a doctor.

If fatty liver is suspected, the doctor probably will order further tests, including a liver-function blood test to measure whether enzymes are elevated (signaling possible liver damage), an ultrasound or a CT scan, and possibly a liver biopsy.

TREATING FATTY LIVER

Although it can be reassuring to hear that most people with simple fatty liver and NAFLD don't develop serious liver problems, it is also estimated that one in four people with NAFLD *will* develop a serious liver disease (NASH) within 10 years. Here are some tips to help manage your NAFLD and NASH:

- **Trim down with diet and exercise.**
  The most effective treatment for fatty liver and the most reliable way to avoid future liver disease result from weight loss and exercise. People with a BMI above 25 can reduce the amount of fat stored in their liver with a diet that is high in fiber and low in calories and saturated fat, but it is important to progress slowly and keep the weight loss to one or two pounds a week.

- **Redistribute the fat.**
  The distribution of body fat can be as important as the BMI in managing NAFLD. Central obesity (visceral fat), the accumulation of a disproportionate amount of weight in the abdomen, puts the individual at high risk for serious liver and heart diseases.

- **Control your diabetes.**
  NAFLD patients with diabetes should begin strict management of the disease to prevent further damage and possibly reduce the liver's fat stores.

- **Control your cholesterol.**
  If cholesterol and triglyceride levels are elevated, diet, exercise, and prescription medications may improve NAFLD.

- **Avoid toxic substances.**
  All patients with NAFLD, especially those diagnosed with NASH, should avoid alcohol, exposure to chemicals that can cause liver damage, cigarette smoke, and those types of herbs that may aggravate liver disease.

BARIATRIC SURGERY

A possible approach to treating nonalcoholic fatty liver disease (NAFLD) may be bariatric surgery, currently the subject of ongoing studies. The Roux-en-Y gastric-bypass procedure (right) connects a small portion of the stomach to a more distal part of the small intestine. Studies have shown that this operation has induced dramatic weight loss and reversed some conditions (such as diabetes) that are risk factors for NAFLD.

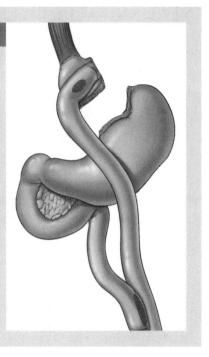

PROSPECTS AND POSSIBILITIES

The prognosis for NAFLD and NASH patients is unclear, though fatty liver alone rarely contributes to a shortening of life span. However, it should be remembered that the metabolic syndrome is made up of several factors that *can* shorten life expectancy. Several ongoing studies supported by the National Institutes of Health and other organizations will better define the natural history of patients with NASH. Still, while one study found that only a tiny percentage of NASH patients develop cirrhosis, another estimated that perhaps 50 percent may eventually develop cirrhosis – especially among patients who fail to control their obesity. Those with NASH who also show iron overload also may be at higher risk for scarring and consequently cirrhosis. Even when cirrhosis has developed, though, there is still every reason to continue adhering to the recommended changes in lifestyle, all of which can contribute to improved quality of life and life expectancy. ◆

Chapter 5

Hemochromatosis

Like so many Americans, Jack took iron supplements almost daily because he thought they gave him an energy boost. His job as a high school English teacher meant spending long nights reading students' papers. He knew that for many of them, he was the last person who would help them build communication skills before they joined the workforce. Jack took that role seriously and when he worked on their papers, he tried hard to give them his full attention.

When he started feeling tired and losing weight, he naturally blamed his late nights. Although he was only 36 years old, he also wasn't surprised when his joints started aching, since he wasn't getting rest or exercising regularly. He decided to get a physical exam and start to put his life more in balance.

During Jack's physical, the doctor asked him whether he took any nutritional supplements. When Jack reported his almost daily doses of iron and mentioned his fatigue and other symptoms, the doctor added bloodwork to the exam, which led to his discovery of Jack's iron overload.

THE MOST COMMON GENETIC DISEASE

One of the great myths of health care in our society is that iron supplements will "pep you up" and harmlessly make you a more energetic person. Few people realize that for those whose blood already is rich in iron, the addition of ferrous sulfate or iron supplements can do severe, irreparable damage to the liver and heart. But why would we be aware of the dangers? Most adults remember television commercials for breakfast cereals, tonics, and pills packed with iron that promised to cure our "iron-poor blood."

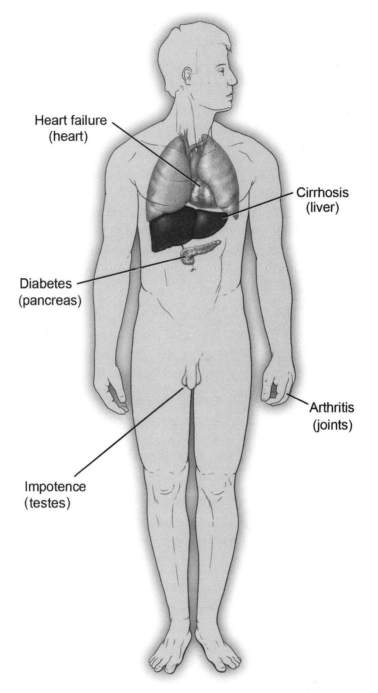

Heart failure
(heart)

Cirrhosis
(liver)

Diabetes
(pancreas)

Arthritis
(joints)

Impotence
(testes)

Hemochromatosis is a hereditary condition characterized by excess iron accumulation in the liver and other vital organs. Untreated, it can result in damage throughout the body, including cirrhosis, diabetes, heart failure, and liver cancer.

Iron supplementation has been a popular remedy for general malaise and fatigue for decades. Yet, because the liver is the body's primary location for storing iron, it suffers the most damage when we have iron overload, a disease called hemochromatosis.

It is true that iron is essential to good health. Iron consumption is essential for people who suffer from iron deficiency anemia or whose iron stores become diminished during pregnancy. Iron is a mineral that helps to form oxygen-carrying hemoglobin in our red blood cells. It boosts brain function, produces energy, and gives us strong muscles and immune systems. We think and feel better when our bodies are getting a healthy supply of iron – small wonder we want more of it!

However, individuals with hereditary hemochromatosis (HH) can experience serious problems if they take in even small amounts of extra iron. Normally, our bodies absorb only about 10 percent of the iron that we consume in food. Most iron circulates in the body in the form of hemoglobin, but some also is stored in the liver, bone marrow, and spleen. People with hemochromatosis, though, can absorb up to 20 percent or more of the iron they take in – twice as much as they need to replace iron lost from the body.

The excess iron is stored first in the liver, but also in the heart, pancreas, joints, pituitary gland, bone marrow, and spleen. Eventually, the iron overload causes the organs to stop working properly, and the patient becomes a candidate for cirrhosis, heart failure, diabetes, and liver cancer.

Eventually, the iron overload causes the organs to stop working properly, and the patient becomes a candidate for cirrhosis, heart failure, diabetes, and liver cancer.

Although hemochromatosis can be caused by other factors as well as genetics, it is the most common genetic disease in the United States – especially among individuals with northern European ancestors such as the Irish, Celtic, British, Scottish, or Nordic peoples – occurring in one in 150 to 200 of this ethnic group. About 1.5 million Americans have the disease, and it is estimated that another 32 million are carriers.

THE GENETIC PUZZLE

Each of us has about 30,000 genes, or information "files," in our chromosomes that determine our development and characteristics. One of these, the HFE gene, helps to control the amount of iron we absorb from food, and carriers of hereditary hemochromatosis have a mutant or altered HFE gene in either a mutation called C282Y or one called H63D. If you inherit a C282Y mutation from one parent, you will be a *carrier* of HH and probably won't develop the disease, though you may absorb some extra iron. In this country, about 10 percent of all Caucasians carry one mutant gene.

Most people with the clinical manifestations of HH such as diabetes, cirrhosis, arthritis, and a type of heart failure have inherited two copies of C282Y – one from each parent – though not all who inherit two C282Y genes go on to develop the clinical form of HH. A few HH patients inherit the two types of mutated genes – one C282Y and one H63D. And quite a few people inherit two H63D genes, though they typically do not go on to develop HH.

Type of Genetic Mutation	Term/Name	Complications
C282Y: One copy	Heterozygote or carrier	None, typically
C282Y: Two copies	Homozygote or true hereditary hemochromatosis	May develop disease
H63D: One copy	Heterozygote	None, typically
H63D: Two copies	Homozygote	None, typically
C282Y and H63D: One copy of each	Compound heterozygote	Possible disease

Complicating the hemochromatosis picture even further are other, rarer forms of the disease, including juvenile hemochromatosis – which carries a high risk of diabetes, irregular heartbeat, heart failure, and gonadal failure, leading to impotence and infertility – and neonatal hemochromatosis, in which iron accumulates in a baby's liver so rapidly that he or she may be stillborn. These conditions, though, are comparatively quite rare.

One group that gets a break with this disease, at least in their younger years, is women, even though the abnormal gene occurs equally in both sexes. Men are at least twice as likely to have iron overload as women, probably because women lose so much iron during menstruation and pregnancy that they store less than men store. The risk for women grows after menopause or a hysterectomy.

HOW DAMAGE HAPPENS

We already mentioned that in keeping us strong, one of iron's tasks is to help build hemoglobin, which carries oxygen throughout the body. Iron's relationship to oxygen is both helpful and harmful, since iron also promotes the creation of free radicals – toxic oxygen molecules that develop in our tissues when we expose our bodies to harmful substances such as cigarette smoke, alcohol, or excessive iron. These free radicals may oxidize molecules in our organs (think of the rust that causes pipes or car bodies to break down and lose their function), corroding them so that they no longer work.

Hemochromatosis may be the slowest-acting of all liver diseases. It can be present in our genes at birth, yet not manifest symptoms until men reach their 40s and women are well into their 50s – and even then, the first symptoms are minor ailments, such as fatigue and joint pain, that don't send most people running to their doctors.

Like many other liver diseases, discomfort in the upper right quadrant of the torso is a symptom. Excessive iron stores in other organs can bring about a noticeable loss of body hair, impotence in men, glucose intolerance, diabetes, and reduced interest in sex. In about 8 percent of patients, the thyroid becomes sluggish (hypothyroidism). At least a quarter of the time, painful joints and arthritis occur, appearing most often in the hands before spreading to the back, neck, and knees.

The most bizarre symptom is a bronze coloration, or hyperpigmentation, that the skin takes on. In fact, hemochromatosis was originally known as "bronze diabetes" because it was in the later stages of the disease, after people developed diabetes symptoms and a grayish-bronze skin tone, that they were diagnosed. Constant thirst and urination generally accompany the skin changes. As hemochromatosis advances, heart irregularities, heart failure, and portal hypertension appear. At that late stage the doctor may also find either an enlarged or a scarred and shrunken liver, shrunken testicles, swollen and tender joints, an enlarged heart, and other signs of cirrhosis.

DIAGNOSING THE ELUSIVE, TREATING THE OBVIOUS

Is there a disorder that *doesn't* involve stiff joints or fatigue?

Hemochromatosis presents a dilemma. The good news is that early detection and treatment can head off the later appearance of life-threatening complications, particularly cirrhosis and liver failure. Yet because the early symptoms are so vague and so common in the population, when people experience them they don't tend to go to the doctor. That is unfortunate, because diagnosing hemochromatosis and treating it early can spare a person the experience of a potentially devastating disease.

But the primary questions remain. Who should be tested for iron overload, and when? First, anyone with a close relative who has been diagnosed with hemochromatosis should certainly be tested. Also, anyone with severe fatigue, heart disease, elevated liver enzymes, impotence, diabetes, or joint disease should have the tests. If your aching joints won't "loosen up" after a two-mile walk, or if you begin your days feeling tired even after a full night's sleep (in other words, if your "ordinary" symptoms begin to seem out of the ordinary), ask your doctor whether tests for hemochromatosis might be appropriate. These include:

- **Serum transferrin saturation.** This test measures the level of iron that is attaching to transferrin, a protein produced in the liver that carries iron in your blood. Transferrin saturation values of more than 45 percent usually indicate a reason for concern and may require further evaluation.

- **Serum ferritin.** This test measures how much iron your body is storing. This test should not be made alone, since many conditions can result in temporarily elevated ferritin levels. If both tests show high numbers, the doctor may want to repeat them after a short time. This test is also used to evaluate a patient's reponse to therapy.

- **A blood test for the HFE gene mutation.**

- **Liver biopsy.** Because of the advances in less invasive diagnostic testing, a liver biopsy is not always needed in order to diagnose hemochromatosis. However, once the diagnosis is made, a biopsy may be performed to measure the amount of iron stored in the liver and the extent of damage caused by iron overload. In cases where the patient is younger than 40 and has normal liver enzymes and a serum ferritin less than 1000, the doctor may decide that the homozygous gene mutation and elevated iron markers in the blood provide sufficient evidence to go ahead with treatment, without the need for a liver biopsy.

- **Sonogram.** The test could show an enlarged liver as well as the presence of liver cancer, especially in patients who already have developed cirrhosis.

- **CT scans and MRIs.** Occasionally, a CT or MRI will further inform the doctor of liver damage or the amount of iron being stored, though a liver biopsy provides much more information.

If caught early enough in the overload process, hemochromatosis can be effectively treated with a "de-ironing" program called phlebotomy. This is a painless regimen of blood removal similar to donating blood and is repeated until your excess iron stores have been depleted.

At first, a pint of blood is removed once or twice a week in a procedure that lasts 30 minutes at most. As your iron levels normalize, your doctor probably will want you to undergo phlebotomy four or five times a year for maintenance. If no organ damage has occurred, phlebotomy usually prevents serious complications such as liver disease, diabetes, and heart disease, and phlebotomy patients have a normal life expectancy. Even if one of those conditions has developed, phlebotomy can slow its progression and even reverse it. When scarring is present in the liver, phlebotomy should be performed at an accelerated rate to prevent cirrhosis.

Once cirrhosis has set in, phlebotomy cannot reverse the damage. It *can* help to preserve liver function and alleviate some symptoms of hemochromatosis (including deep fatigue) so that cirrhosis patients can more comfortably cope with their disease.

Phlebotomy can even resolve the bronze skin coloration caused by hemochromatosis, and it can improve congestive heart failure caused by hemochromatosis.

Phlebotomy won't resolve all conditions caused by the hemochromatosis. About half the people with diabetes will see an improvement in the control of that condition. It usually will not reverse hemochromatosis-related impotence. Arthritis and joint pain will usually continue, and patients should exercise caution when treating that pain with nonsteroidal anti-inflammatories (NSAIDs, ibuprofen-like drugs), because these medications can aggravate liver damage, cause ulcers, and adversely affect the kidneys.

Dietary restrictions are not emphasized in maintaining proper levels of iron because phlebotomy is so effective at ridding the body of excessive iron. Nonetheless, patients should refrain from taking multivitamin preparations with added iron as well as vitamin C supplements (including multivitamins containing C), because vitamin C helps the body absorb iron from food. Cereals fortified with iron should be avoided and so should some herbal supplements that are popular in treating liver disease (including milk thistle, dandelion, and licorice) if they contain iron. Needless to say, hemochromatosis patients learn to become expert readers of product labels.

Alcohol, too, should be avoided. In combination with excessive iron it is particularly toxic to the liver; one study showed that hemochromatosis patients who drank even moderate amounts of alcohol every day were nine times as likely to contract cirrhosis and liver cancer as those who drank little or not at all.

The long-term prognosis is good for hemochromatosis patients like Jack, who had not developed extensive organ damage and had resolved to find balance and create a healthier lifestyle for himself on all fronts. With proper preventive treatment and phlebotomy, they can expect to live normal, active, and full lives. Furthermore, with the routine availability of simple iron tests and the gene mutation test, the risk to Jack's immediate relatives (siblings and children) can also be assessed and they can be treated, if necessary. ◆

Chapter 6

Wilson Disease

At 17, Jessica was a typical teenager – most of the time. Active in her school's choir and drama clubs, Jessica kept busy on weekends with homework and parties.

For several years, however, she had been developing psychiatric symptoms that seemed to come out of nowhere. Her behaviors ranged from a dark, enraged silence to uncontrollable grinning at inappropriate times. At times, she slurred her words and seemed clumsy. As Jessica's behavior became progressively worse, her parents suspected drug and alcohol abuse, though that seemed out of character for their daughter.

Jessica's grades plummeted. Sharing her parents' deep concern for the girl, her teachers recommended that she see a psychiatrist. That doctor diagnosed her with depression and prescribed an antidepressant. Although her behavior seemed to stabilize for a short while, Jessica noticed that her eyes and skin were yellowing slightly. After a few weeks, she started complaining about a dull ache in her abdomen.

Her parents, too, had noticed the beginning of jaundice. They were alarmed – jaundice is a symptom that is widely associated with liver disease. They made an immediate appointment for their daughter to see a liver specialist, and the mystery surrounding young Jessica's symptoms was about to be solved.

To the family's surprise, the liver doctor referred Jessica to an eye specialist, an ophthalmologist, to examine her for evidence of "K-F rings" – the rings around her corneas that indicate Wilson disease (WD).

Tests showed that Jessica's jaundice and stomach pain as well as her nervous symptoms indeed had been brought on by Wilson disease, but fortunately it was discovered before it caused extensive damage to the liver or her nervous system. She will have to follow a strict regimen of medication for the rest of her life, but if she monitors her condition carefully, Jessica should be able to lead a normal life.

WHAT IS WILSON DISEASE?

In the way it behaves, WD might seem to be the most straightforward of all liver diseases. Simply put, it develops when the genetic abnormality that primarily affects the function of the liver leads to copper accumulation in the body, first in the liver, then in other organs, especially the brain, eyes, and kidneys.

This happens because of a rare occurrence. Wilson disease is inherited as an autosomal recessive trait, meaning that the patient must receive two copies of the same abnormal gene, one from each parent, before the disease can occur. Because of that, WD is an extremely rare disorder: Only one of 30,000 to 50,000 people will be diagnosed with it. (People who inherit only one of the abnormal genes are carriers of the disease but are not afflicted with it.)

The two abnormal inherited genes work together to create a disorder of copper metabolism, meaning that the liver cannot metabolize copper or process it properly, which causes accumulation of copper in the body to rise to dangerous levels. No one is sure exactly what causes the "Wilson gene" (actually the ATP7B gene, located on the long arm of chromosome 13) to mutate. We know what it *should* be doing before it mutates; the ATP7B gene regulates a protein that helps transport copper in bile out of the liver.

Scientists used to think that the important abnormality people with WD displayed was that they were not able to produce enough ceruloplasmin, an enzyme in the blood that binds to copper and helps to regulate and transport it. Now it is understood that the reduction in ceruloplasmin is a result of the liver's inability to metabolize copper, rather than its cause. All the evidence points to diminished excretion of copper by the biliary system, the result of the abnormal ATP7B protein produced by the mutated WD gene.

We do know that copper is necessary in our bodies. We need it for many important body enzymes and proteins. Copper is needed for the proteins that make us grow, it helps our nerves function effectively, and it helps control inflammation and damage caused by free radicals.

The symptoms that make up Wilson disease – tremors, rigidity, slow movements – were noticed as a group as early as 1883. In 1890, researchers discovered a connection between liver cirrhosis and brain changes; later, two physicians would add golden-brown rings (known as "Kayser-Fleischer rings") around the cornea to the list of signs in this grouping.

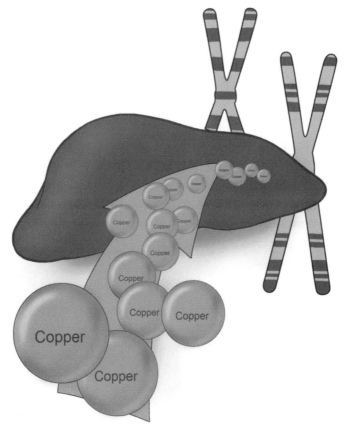

In Wilson disease, a disorder of copper metabolism caused by abnormal genes, excessive accumulation of copper in the body can rise to dangerous levels, causing cirrhosis and psychiatric problems.

Finally, in 1912, Samuel A. Kinnear Wilson connected some of the dots.

Born in New Jersey, Wilson was raised and educated in Edinburgh, Scotland. After graduating from medical school, he became house physician at the Royal Edinburgh Infirmary, where his lifelong fascination with neurology began. He went on to practice, teach, and continue research in London, where his patients included the legendary film star Charlie Chaplin.

In research conducted while he was still a resident in training, Wilson noticed that this peculiar set of symptoms and signs – the lack of physical coordination, personality changes, and K-F rings – developed in young people and that most of the patients died within five years of the onset of symptoms. While cirrhosis was found consistently during autopsies, these young patients had not necessarily exhibited symptoms of cirrhosis when they were alive. This variety of cirrhosis was not related to alcohol, but inflammation, fatty degeneration, and scarring were present in their livers.

CLINICAL PICTURE OF WILSON DISEASE

For patients with Wilson disease, copper buildup begins at birth, when abnormal liver function fails to enable excretion of sufficient copper. Symptoms can appear when patients are as young as 6 years of age, but usually the effects aren't noticeable until the teen years. As we saw with Jessica in our earlier example, they may experience abdominal pain and swelling, jaundice, or other symptoms connected with the diseased liver.

If the condition is not treated, the liver will reach and exceed its capacity to store copper, and copper will begin to accumulate in other organs, especially the brain. At that point, symptoms will become more pronounced and include difficulties with speech, writing, walking, and swallowing. There may be psychiatric problems such as depression, suicidal tendencies, dementia, severe insomnia, and inability to focus. A low blood count can result as copper accumulates throughout the body. A golden-brown pigmentation, the Kayser-Fleischer rings, can develop in the eyes. Abnormal twisting of the body and slowness of movements, especially in the tongue, lips, fingers, and jaw, can occur, along with involuntary tremors and drooling.

In extreme cases, kidneys can lose their function. Some patients might have extremely low levels of circulating hemoglobin and blood platelets, leading to bruising and bleeding. Joint problems can develop with degeneration of the joints.

At these later stages, Wilson disease resembles many other illnesses. Fortunately, diagnosing WD today is relatively straightforward, so there is little reason for the disease to progress to its dangerous stages.

DIAGNOSING WILSON DISEASE

With the early symptoms – abdominal discomfort or swelling, possible jaundice – so clearly pointing to liver involvement, most physicians who see these symptoms in a person under 20 years old would take care to exclude Wilson disease. A reliable diagnosis would require several tests.

The first diagnostic test would measure the level of serum ceruloplasmin, a copper-binding protein in the blood. In 95 percent of patients with Wilson disease, levels of this protein are lower than normal.

Doctors also would measure urinary copper excretion over a 24-hour period. In most Wilson patients displaying other symptoms, copper excretion levels are unusually high.

Patients also might undergo a slit-lamp examination, a special eye exam used to confirm the presence of Kayser-Fleischer rings, the golden- or greenish-brown rings around the corneas. These rings are present in about 50 percent of Wilson patients.

Finally, the physician might order a liver biopsy to measure the amount of copper in the liver. The patient's family might also be asked to undergo the less invasive screenings for the disease even if they exhibit no symptoms.

In fact, because most cases of Wilson disease are passed down through the generations, physicians increasingly view genetic testing for siblings as a necessity rather than a mere precaution. With genetic testing, family members can be treated for Wilson before they become ill. The standard test for genetic diagnosis is a blood test known as "haplotype analysis," with actual gene tests already around the corner.

Researchers across North America are learning more about WD every day. Their work is taking them in several directions; two of the most exciting approaches are prenatal genetic testing and drugs that might actually lower the copper levels in the body. The latter approach is already a reality.

TREATING WILSON DISEASE: THE OUTLOOK IS GOOD

For past generations, Wilson disease was invariably fatal, because there was no way to remove excess copper from the system. Today, the outlook for Wilson patients is most positive: Drug therapy extracts accumulated body copper and prevents future buildup.

The first step is chelation therapy – that is, the use of drugs that will remove excessive copper from the liver and other organs. The most common chelating drug is D-penicillamine, sold under the trade names of Cuprimine and Depen. D-penicillamine binds to copper and expels it through the kidneys into the urine.

Unfortunately, this medicine has a number of side effects. D-penicillamine tends to deplete the body of vitamin B_6, so it's important that the patient take supplements during chelation. Other complications to watch for include rash, fever, swelling of lymph nodes, low levels of circulating platelets or white blood cells, protein in the urine, or development of serious illnesses such as systemic lupus erythematosus, myasthenia gravis, or aplastic anemia. Typically, D-penicillamine is prescribed in small doses at first, then in gradually increasing amounts.

When complications arise, the physician might prescribe other chelating drugs, including trientine (marketed as Syprine) or tetrathiomolybdate, which have fewer serious side effects.

Once chelation therapy has achieved removal of most of the excess copper, WD patients need to prevent future reaccumulation with maintenance therapy. For most patients, zinc acetate (or gluconate) taken by mouth blocks the absorption of copper by the intestines and promotes its elimination in the stool. Zinc acetate also helps stimulate the production of metallothionein, which binds copper in the intestine and keeps it from passing on to the liver or other organs.

Further measures are required for WD patients. For them, lifelong maintenance does not stop with drugs and vitamin B_6 supplements. It is important for them to avoid copper intake even in the foods they eat – though it would be impossible to avoid copper altogether, since it is present in small amounts in many foods. They can, however, help ensure healthy livers by not eating foods that are particularly copper-rich; those include cocoa, chocolate, liver, mushrooms, nuts, shellfish, and sardines. And, like patients who contract any liver disease, WD patients should not drink alcohol. Most important, though, is one recommendation that cannot be emphasized enough: WD patients should not discontinue their medicine just because they are feeling so much better. If they should do so, copper will reaccumulate and their livers are at high risk of failing completely.

In cases where Wilson disease has caused irreversible liver damage or acute liver failure, or for those few individuals who do not respond to chelation therapy, a liver transplant is an important and life-saving option. Transplantation effectively cures Wilson disease, and the long-term survival rate following the transplant is about 80 percent. Early diagnosis and chelation, however, followed by faithful maintenance, heads off the need to consider a transplant for the vast majority of patients with Wilson disease. ◆

Chapter 7

Alcoholic Liver Disease

There is a "good drinker" in every group of friends, that one individual who can put away more alcohol than anyone else in the crowd but never seems to get obnoxiously drunk.

Jerry, an attorney in his mid-40s, was one of those "good" drinkers. He would meet three or four other lawyers for drinks at a popular downtown bar at least twice a week. Even after three or four martinis, Jerry never stumbled or slurred his words. Whether he and his girlfriend met for dinner or he was at home alone, relaxing in front of the television, Jerry usually enjoyed several glasses of wine. Most days, Jerry sipped four or five drinks over the course of the evening. But he always was more or less sober, so his alcohol consumption wasn't a problem. Or so he thought.

The first symptom he noticed was a diminished sexual drive – not that Jerry would have guessed that his libido could be connected to a liver problem – and, soon after, a growing fatigue. As a supposedly healthy and relatively young man, he knew that both symptoms were unusual. Since Jerry had never admitted to himself that he had a drinking problem, his doctor had to run a battery of blood tests, as well as question Jerry at length about his drinking habits, before alcoholic liver disease, or ALD, finally was diagnosed. Fortunately, Jerry's ALD had not progressed to cirrhosis, and he agreed to abstain from alcohol completely and permanently. If he honors that agreement, Jerry can expect more than a 90 percent chance of living a normal life.

A SOCIETAL DISORDER

Considering the extensive use of alcohol in our society, it should come as no surprise that an estimated 10 percent of American adults experience an alcohol-related disease. Liquor is easily accessible, it is inexpensive, and it is seen by many as a necessary part of socializing. When one individual in a group prefers water or soda to an alcoholic drink, it is almost inevitable that someone will try to persuade the nondrinker to switch to beer or wine. Without alcohol, in fact, it is difficult for many people to plan a party or other social event, though most people are aware that when abused, alcohol is a toxic substance.

Those social pressures have resulted in a diagnosis of alcoholic liver disease (ALD) for about 25 percent of adults with alcohol-related diseases. Often leading to more serious liver damage, ALD has become one of the most common causes of death for middle-aged adults in America; moreover, ALD is an equal-opportunity disease, found among men and women of every economic, racial, and social background.

ALCOHOL AND THE LIVER

To appreciate the consequences of ALD, one needs to understand how alcohol affects the liver.

The liver works to protect our bodies from all harmful substances. When we drink alcohol, the liver metabolizes it, breaking it down into less dangerous substances so that it won't build up in our bloodstreams. In most instances, the liver recruits enzymes, or proteins known as alcohol dehydrogenase and aldehyde dehydrogenase, to transform the alcohol into a harmless product.

There also is a system of special-duty enzymes within the liver, known as the cytochrome P-450 system, which converts certain fat-soluble materials into water-soluble substances so that they can be processed and excreted as waste. Unfortunately, alcohol is both water-soluble and fat-soluble, so it is adept at permeating other organs and damaging them. And when both enzyme systems fail to work correctly – or if they are suppressed by the sheer volume of alcohol entering the body – then the liver and other organs inevitably are damaged.

HOW ALD DEVELOPS

Because only one-fourth of all alcoholics are diagnosed with ALD, we know that other contributing factors are important in leading to development of liver disease. Of course, patients who consume great quantities of liquor and maintain their heavy drinking for years are most at risk for ALD.

However, it is the quantity of *alcohol* itself, rather than the number of drinks consumed, that puts a person at risk. For instance, the individual who drank six wine spritzers every evening for five years would be at a smaller risk of contracting ALD than someone who drank six glasses of undiluted wine, and certainly the risk for the spritzer drinker would be dramatically lower than for someone who drank a liter of whiskey each day.

According to the rule of thumb, consumption of 80 grams of alcohol every day – about a six-pack of beer or a liter of wine – is the threshold of possibility for men to develop ALD. Women are more vulnerable to the damaging effects of alcohol, and they would need to ingest only about 20 grams of alcohol per day to lead to a likelihood of ALD. These levels of consumption would have to be sustained over long periods; no one is quite sure how long it takes for ALD to develop, but at this pace cirrhosis can develop in just five years.

Genetics also plays a part in whether ALD occurs. Ironically, it is those individuals like Jerry, our "good drinker," who are most likely to develop ALD. The person we think of as a "good drinker" actually metabolizes alcohol more quickly than other drinkers and therefore would have to drink more in order to feel the same effects from the liquor. This "ability to hold liquor" has a genetic basis. Individuals who have been drinking heavily and consistently for many years are at higher risk for liver damage.

Another genetic factor connected with alcohol and the liver occurs in many Asians. For some unknown reason, one of the alcohol-metabolizing enzymes, aldehyde dehydrogenase, is faulty and allows a chemical, acetaldehyde, to gather in the bodies of Asians when they drink any alcohol at all, causing severe nausea, flushing, and an accelerated heart rate. For this reason, many Asians find consumption of any alcohol at all quite intolerable.

As noted above, women have a lower alcohol tolerance than men do. Perhaps because of this, women often contract ALD and cirrhosis at a younger age than men do. It also has been found that women with alcohol-based cirrhosis will have a shorter life expectancy than their male counterparts. While lower body weight and hormonal differences are sometimes assumed to be the cause of this imbalance, the more likely factor is that many women have a lesser amount of the enzyme alcohol dehydrogenase in their bodies; therefore they do not metabolize alcohol as well as men do.

Interestingly, it also has been shown that women seek help for their alcoholism and alcohol-related problems only half as often as men do, and they may be better at hiding their addictions until the liver has been damaged.

It also has been found that alcohol toxicity levels can be affected by the interaction between drugs and alcohol. In an ALD patient who is actively drinking, ingesting as little as 4 grams (only 8 extra-strength tablets) of acetaminophen (Tylenol) in one 24-hour period may cause serious liver damage – though it is also true that a relatively small dose of acetaminophen (2 grams per day) may be safer for liver patients than the use of aspirin or NSAIDs such as Motrin or generic ibuprofen. The smallest doses of aspirin or ibuprofen can be harmful to ALD patients, causing bleeding and kidney disorders.

Alcohol may also amplify side effects of many drugs. Taken with cimetidine (Tagamet) or ranitidine (Zantac), alcohol can affect levels of these and other medications in the blood and influence their effectiveness. Mixing alcohol and any pain reliever or medication, even over-the-counter pills, can be dangerous; always check with a physician or pharmacist beforehand.

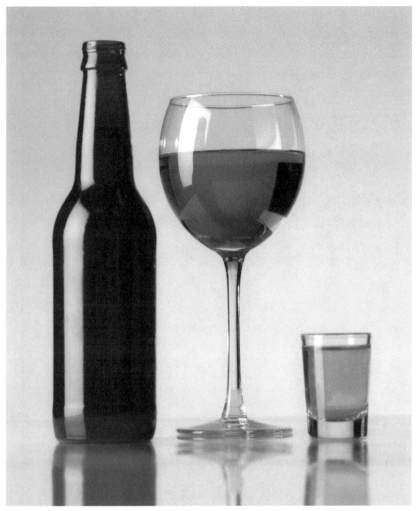

Alcohol equivalents: *A standard 12-ounce bottle of American beer (about 5 percent alcohol) is equal to a 5-ounce glass of wine (12 percent alcohol) or 1.5 ounces of hard liquor (40 percent alcohol or 80-proof spirits).*

Other factors that might not seem harmful to the liver at first glance can greatly affect the progression of ALD. Malnutrition, specifically a shortage of calories and protein in the diet, is common among ALD patients, as are vitamin and mineral deficiencies. Obesity, too, influences ALD: Overweight patients with ALD are at higher risk for developing cirrhosis than are ALD patients of normal weight, so it is important for those with ALD to maintain their diet and exercise regimens.

Lastly, ALD patients with diabetes are at greater risk for cirrhosis than those with consistently normal blood-sugar levels. ALD patients who already have diabetes often need medications to control their blood-sugar levels.

DETECTING ALD

As with many liver diseases, the outward symptoms of ALD are vague and shared with a wide variety of disorders. Fatigue and weakness are the most common symptoms; infertility and a decrease in sexual desire or function also may be present. Insomnia, difficulty concentrating, depression, tremors, and emotional problems can be other indicators.

Physically, the patient might develop an enlarged liver or spleen, muscular or testicular atrophy – a result of a shift in the patient's estrogen balance – or spider angiomatas.

As the doctor notes these inconclusive symptoms, the most important diagnostic tool may be the doctor's ability to elicit details of the patient's drinking habits and to recognize possible denial of a drink-

THE CAGE QUESTIONNAIRE

This simple test takes only a minute to answer and may help you and your doctor determine whether you need to look more closely at your drinking behavior.

- Have you ever felt that you needed to *cut down* on your drinking?
- Have people *annoyed* you by criticizing your drinking?
- Have you ever felt *guilty* about drinking?
- Have you ever felt that you needed a drink first thing in the morning (*eye-opener*) to steady your nerves or get rid of a hangover?

If you answered "yes" to two or more questions, it is time to talk to your doctor about the impact your drinking may have on your health.

ing problem. The doctor might also detect alcohol on the patient's breath – an important observation, particularly for a patient attending a daytime appointment!

One important clue to a hidden alcohol problem can be found in the patient's answers to the CAGE Questionnaire (see page 76). It also can be important for the doctor to meet with the family members closest to the patient. This is a delicate and sensitive situation, requiring considerable skill and experience.

If ALD is suspected, several blood tests can support the diagnosis. While there is no one blood test that can definitively point to a diagnosis of ALD, the combined results of several tests can aid the physician's findings, especially in cases where the patient is not forthcoming with personal information or is in denial.

It is helpful, first, to measure a routine blood count (high MCV, i.e., red-cell volume) and the liver enzymes. The enzyme GGTP usually is elevated in patients with ALD (though the same elevations also will be found in other liver diseases). The transaminases AST and ALT also may be higher than normal, with the AST often measuring two or three times higher than the ALT, possibly due to a vitamin B$_6$ deficiency common among alcoholics.

The blood-alcohol level also should be tested, though these tests indicate only alcohol drunk in the previous 24 hours and may not be a clue to the patient's ongoing drinking habits. Uric acid levels and triglyceride levels also may be high in people with ALD, while zinc, magnesium, phosphorus, and potassium levels can be low. The doctor may also find a thyroid disorder and vitamin deficiencies (pointing to poor nutrition, common among very heavy drinkers). Again, none of these indicators alone would be confirmation of a diagnosis of ALD, but when they are present in clusters, they are important clues.

If the physician runs a sonogram or a CT scan, a fatty liver could be an additional pointer, as could an enlarged spleen or liver.

When the above tests lead to a diagnosis of ALD, a liver biopsy often confirms the diagnosis and pinpoints the extent of liver damage and the stage of the disease, enabling the doctor to make an informed prognostic evaluation.

THE PROGRESSION OF ALD

ALD is found in three distinct stages: alcoholic fatty liver, alcoholic hepatitis, and alcoholic cirrhosis. Symptoms felt by the patient may not differ significantly among the stages, and since the first two stages (fatty liver and alcoholic hepatitis) can be reversed, it is important to determine exactly how far the disease has progressed. The only test that can reliably provide that information is a liver biopsy.

A fatty liver, or steatosis, can develop after just a few days of heavy drinking. Many "weekend drinkers" or "vacation drinkers" may have developed fatty liver at some point in their lives, though they probably experienced no symptoms. Alcoholic fatty liver almost always is reversible when the alcohol intake ceases, with no serious consequences.

Alcoholic hepatitis, however, is a more serious inflammation of the liver caused by alcohol toxicity, and it also may be asymptomatic. If there are no symptoms, the alcoholic hepatitis probably would be found during a routine blood test, when abnormal LFTs appear. This patient's condition, too, is reversible if he or she stops drinking alcohol immediately.

However, many patients with alcoholic hepatitis become seriously ill, and for them the disease can be fatal. Their symptoms can include fever, nausea, vomiting, and liver failure; if they survive, it may take them many months to recover. Those who continue drinking alcohol have as much as a 50 percent chance of developing cirrhosis within 10 years, but if they stop drinking permanently, they may be able to restore their good liver health.

Alcoholic cirrhosis, the last stage of ALD, means that alcohol has caused severe scarring of the liver, and it can lead to the same complications found in other forms of cirrhosis. Once those complications develop, the alcoholic cirrhosis cannot be reversed; the liver will not return to normal. Further, alcoholic cirrhosis patients have about a 15 percent chance of developing liver cancer over the following years, despite abstinence from alcohol.

TREATING ALD

For the early and mid-stages of ALD, one treatment is supremely effective: The total and permanent cessation of alcohol consumption may restore the liver to total normality.

Along with a commitment to sobriety, support programs such as AA (Alcoholics Anonymous) have proved immensely helpful to millions of recovering alcoholics over the years. Family, friends, and co-workers of the alcoholic may also find meaningful support in Al-Anon, a related 12-step program.

It also is important that the newly sober ALD patient rebuild his or her health with a program of sound nutrition and exercise. Information on how to become healthier and stronger is ubiquitous; one can walk into any bookstore or newsstand and find thousands of resources. To help readers start planning a healthier future, Chapter 17 of this book includes basic nutrition and exercise guidelines.

For those with more severe alcoholic hepatitis (the third stage described above), there are several medicine-based treatments to consider as well. Corticosteroids, or anti-inflammatory medications, can boost the chances for survival in patients with severe alcoholic hepatitis. Prednisone and other corticosteroids do carry side effects, so they are not recommended as long-term treatment, but are reserved for those with bad prognostic indicators of severe and potentially life-threatening disease.

Another treatment often recommended is the use of antioxidants to help enhance the liver's protection against alcohol and other toxins, as well as a daily vitamin and mineral regimen to replenish what may have been depleted during the patient's illness and poor nutrition.

With complete abstinence and good nutrition, the prognosis for most ALD patients is positive, especially if alcohol intake ceases before the onset of cirrhosis. If the ALD does not progress to the cirrhosis stage, the inflammation and liver damage caused by ALD has the potential to be reversible: Statistics show that 90 percent of those patients will experience a good quality of life at a rate only slightly below that of the non-ALD population. Even after cirrhosis is discovered, patients who abstain from alcohol have a greater chance of better survival in good health, so it is never too late to adopt a better lifestyle.

WHEN ALD IS MORE THAN ALD

It's worth noting that alcohol not only causes ALD, it also hastens the progression of many other liver diseases. Alcohol is toxic to the liver, and if any liver disease is suspected, alcohol consumption should stop immediately.

Three liver diseases are particularly susceptible to alcohol and its damaging effects:

- **Hepatitis C.** Studies have shown that alcohol triggers the replication, multiplication, and ill effects of the hepatitis C virus (HCV). Even worse, for patients with chronic HCV, drinking even small amounts of alcohol can hasten the advance of cirrhosis.

- **Hepatitis B.** The hepatitis B virus (HBV) is found to be active more often in alcoholics than in the general population and very often in ALD patients with cirrhosis. In ALD patients, the HBV infection is likely to be much more serious than the same infection in non-ALD patients – another reason that abstinence from alcohol is so important for people with ALD.

- **Hemochromatosis.** Alcohol can enhance iron toxicity, so patients with hemochromatosis and other iron-overload diseases risk additional liver damage if they continue drinking. ◆

Chapter 8

Primary Biliary Cirrhosis

Helga's name implied a certain kind of woman, and she always had believed that image of herself: sturdy, in control of things, a hard worker and good mother. So as she reached her late 50s, Helga was surprised to feel herself slowing down. She felt tired almost every day, and for the first time in her life, she started needing naps – sometimes before noon. Helga also was distressed to be diagnosed with early osteoporosis, a disorder common in postmenopausal women that causes the bones to become porous and brittle.

Helga soon developed a symptom that was almost more annoying than her fatigue. She itched. The itching, or pruritus, was on her legs, her arms, her stomach, and her back. She ruled out the elastic in her clothes as the cause, because many of the itchiest places never touched elastic. A friend suggested that Helga see a dermatologist; it sounded like a good idea, but he, too, was baffled – until she mentioned her serious fatigue. "It's really starting to depress me," she said. "Feeling tired all the time makes me just want to give up. I think it's even giving me a chronic stomachache."

Helga's depression, fatigue, and stomach discomfort, coupled with her pruritus, gave the dermatologist a clue to her ailment.

Helga's depression, fatigue, and stomach discomfort, coupled with her pruritus, gave the dermatologist a clue to her ailment. He referred her to a liver specialist, who quickly diagnosed her problem: primary biliary cirrhosis (PBC), an incurable but very treatable inflammatory disease of the liver.

WHAT IS PBC?

Primary biliary cirrhosis is a disease that attacks the small, intrahepatic (inside the liver) bile ducts. It is a particularly gradual disease with a very slow progression; life for the patient is virtually normal for more than 20 years. However, in its later course PBC produces more than just abnormal liver tests. At this stage symptoms and signs develop. Ideally, it is better for the disease to be diagnosed in the stage occurring before symptoms arise, so that treatment to slow its progression may be initiated.

PBC is an autoimmune disease, which puts it in the same "family" as more familiar autoimmune diseases such as thyroid disorders, lupus, rheumatoid arthritis, and autoimmune hepatitis, in which the immune system attacks the liver's cells. With PBC, the targets for the inflammation are the cells of the bile ducts, with later spillage of the inflammation farther into the liver, causing its eventual scarring (cirrhosis). For most PBC patients, the term "cirrhosis" is quite premature, as the amount of scarring is quite minor.

Although PBC occurs worldwide, it is seen most often in Caucasians from northern Europe. It sometimes runs in families; parents, siblings, and children of PBC patients are far more likely than the general population to be diagnosed with PBC. More than 90 percent of PBC patients are women, and while women under 30 and over 90 years of age have been diagnosed with PBC, most often it is found in women between the ages of 40 and 60.

While research has identified those geographic-, gender-, and age-based associations, the exact cause of PBC remains unknown. Because of its frequency in certain parts of the world, scientists suspect environmental factors as possible PBC triggers, if not actual causes. Some that have already been investigated include contaminated well water, cigarette smoking, viruses, bacteria, nail polish, and even substances such as estrogen, interferon, or chlorpromazine, an antipsychotic drug.

Infections, too, have been suspected as causes of the disease. The herpes virus that causes shingles is being studied, as are E. coli, the

Epstein-Barr virus, mycobacteria (similar to the bacteria that cause tuberculosis), chlamydia pneumonia, and HIV-1, a virus similar to the one that causes AIDS.

HOW IS PBC DIAGNOSED?

As we saw in Helga's case, the most common symptoms of PBC would not necessarily indicate possible liver disease unless they are viewed together. In fact, more than half the patients diagnosed with PBC display no symptoms at all; for them, an elevated alkaline phosphatase (AP) obtained during routine blood tests may lead to further testing and the discovery of the antibody present in PBC, the antimitochondrial antibody (AMA). It is presumed, however, that most patients with a positive AMA will eventually develop symptomatic PBC, but it may take up to 10 years to surface.

Fatigue is the most common symptom, reported by about two-thirds of PBC patients. Pruritus also is exceedingly common, manifesting in more than half of PBC cases. Unexplained weight loss, depression, sleep disorders, abdominal pain, urinary tract infections, and joint pain often accompany the itching and fatigue. In more advanced cases, the skin may darken with excess deposits of a pigment called melanin, and the liver might be tender. In rare cases, finger clubbing – enlarged, rounded fingertips – also may be a sign of PBC.

In about 20 percent of PBC cases, flat, fatty yellow plaques called xanthelasmas (occurring around the eyes) and more nodular xanthomas (found in creases of the legs, hands, and arms, or on joints) are seen as physical signs. Both these signs are related to an elevated cholesterol that accompanies the disease. Several medications can be prescribed to shrink the nodules, albeit with variable results. The good news is that the elevated cholesterol does not appear to cause a significant increase in coronary artery disease.

Diagnosing PBC usually calls for a combination of approaches, starting with laboratory testing. Doctors generally look for a pattern of blood abnormalities known as intrahepatic cholestasis, as well as the AMA. About 95 percent of PBC patients test positive for AMA, so it is a fairly reliable indicator of PBC. The antibody immunoglobulin M (IgM) also is usually elevated in PBC patients.

When PBC is suspected, a liver biopsy may be needed to assess the damage done to the liver thus far and to determine how far the disease may have progressed. PBC develops in four stages, and only a liver biopsy can tell doctors which stage is current and how to proceed with treatment:

- **Stage 1** reveals damage to the bile ducts, and granulomas (tiny microscopic nodules filled with inflammatory cells) often are present.

- **Stage 2** shows inflammation beyond the bile ducts and the formation of tiny new ductules rather like twigs sprouting from the branches of a tree.

- **Stage 3** indicates that fibrosis (scarring) has become noticeable.

- **Stage 4** is the most advanced stage, with cirrhosis present.

Progress through the various stages is unpredictable. Some people progress quickly through Stage 1, then remain in Stage 2 for a decade, while others will linger in Stage 1 for years before they move through Stage 2 to Stage 3.

PBC'S PARTNERS IN CRIME

The following conditions all may be associated with PBC:

- Vitiligo
- Fatigue
- Depression
- Raynaud's phenomenon
- Gallstones
- Osteoporosis
- Hypothyroidism
- Sjögren's syndrome
- Scleroderma
- Lupus
- Vitamin A deficiency
- Vitamin D deficiency
- Vitamin E deficiency
- Vitamin K deficiency

The list of disorders that may be associated with PBC is lengthy and diverse; it is a disease that shares the disorders associated with many other systems. One of the most common is thyroid disease, usually hypothyroidism (underactive thyroid). About 20 percent of PBC patients have some thyroid dysfunction, and the two illnesses share some symptoms, including fatigue and depression. Often, treating the hypothyroidism with medication helps immensely in addressing PBC patients' fatigue.

Rheumatologic disorders (connective-tissue disorders) are also autoimmune-related. Of these, one of the most common among PBC patients is Sjögren's syndrome, indicated by dry eyes and mouth, and sometimes by trouble swallowing.

Other examples are scleroderma, a hardening and thickening of the skin that can sometimes be present in PBC patients, and rheumatoid arthritis, characterized by joint pain and later joint deformities; Raynaud's phenomenon, in which fingertips become numb and blue in cold temperatures; and systemic lupus erythematosus, in which the patient suffers from fever, skin rash, and arthritis.

The skin is affected by PBC, causing not only pruritus and xanthomas, but on occasion vitiligo, characterized by smooth, colorless patches all over the body. Kidney disorders, especially urinary tract infections, affect one-fifth of all female PBC patients, and sarcoidosis – the formation of granulomas in the liver, bones, lymph nodes, skin, and lungs – sometimes accompanies PBC as well. Gallstones, diarrhea, and abdominal pain all are common with PBC; in fact, nearly 40 percent of PBC patients may develop gallstones.

Osteoporosis is frequently seen in PBC patients. Deficiencies in fat-soluble vitamins also are problematic because they can be absorbed only with fats and bile, and the bile delivery system is seriously impaired in PBC. Consequently, patients may be deficient in vitamins A, D, E, and K – and without sufficient vitamin D, calcium is not absorbed well, possibly contributing to osteoporosis in PBC patients. Their best approach is to talk to their doctors about which nutritional supplements they should be taking.

IT CAN'T BE CURED,
BUT IT CAN BE TREATED

Because there is no cure for PBC, and because the speed at which it progresses cannot be predicted, all PBC treatments are geared to controlling the symptoms and slowing the disease.

Several medications that have been studied in treating PBC are not often prescribed because of their negative side effects, including the steroid prednisone, which can contribute to PBC-related bone loss; cyclosporine, which can cause high blood pressure and impair kidney function; and chlorambucil, a chemotherapy drug that might damage bone marrow. At this writing, only one medication appears to be helpful in treating PBC: ursodeoxycholic acid.

Ursodeoxycholic acid (UDCA) is the most popular drug for treating PBC and the only medication approved by the FDA for this use.

Ursodeoxycholic acid (UDCA) is the most popular drug for treating PBC and the only medication approved by the FDA for this use. Originally developed to dissolve gallstones, UDCA is a natural bile acid that is not toxic to the liver. It has been found to be protective to the liver, delaying and preventing the destruction of bile ducts, thus delaying the progression of PBC to cirrhosis. Individuals taking UDCA show significant improvement in their liver function and cholesterol tests. In some cases, UDCA combats symptoms such as fatigue and itching, so that not only are the lives of patients prolonged with this drug, but they also enjoy a higher quality of life with very few side effects.

While UDCA helps to ease the symptoms or slow the progression of PBC, the disease may eventually advance to cirrhosis, with worsening tests signaling the possible need for a liver transplant. Once the transplant is performed, the long-term prognosis is excellent. Even if PBC recurs in the new liver, which happens in a few cases, the progression of the disease is slow and the patient can experience a good quality of life for decades.

WHAT IS THE PROGNOSIS
FOR PBC PATIENTS?

Patients may live for many years after their initial diagnoses, particularly when the disease is slowed by effective modern therapy and appropriate nutritional supplements. Moreover, there are effective treatments to control pruritus (itching), a very distressing symptom for many people.

A mathematical model, known as the Mayo PBC Model, can predict survival based on lab results and clinical features, and can determine when a liver transplant is needed. (For more information on the Mayo PBC model, go to http://www.mayoclinic.org/girst/mayomodel1.html.)

It should be noted, too, that three other liver diseases may closely resemble PBC in many features: autoimmune cholangitis and primary sclerosing cholangitis, both covered in other chapters of this book, and PBC with autoimmune features, or "overlap syndrome." Nearly 12 percent of PBC patients are diagnosed with overlap syndrome, which means that they have features of both PBC and autoimmune hepatitis.

Because the treatment and prognosis may be quite different for patients with these diseases, it is important that patients obtain the most precise diagnosis and receive the most appropriate treatment plan possible. ◆

Chapter 9

Primary Sclerosing Cholangitis

When Ben started itching, it didn't occur to him that he might be on the brink of a serious health challenge. A fairly fit 43-year-old accountant, Ben tried to eat sensibly and jogged or lifted weights at least four times a week. Beyond an occasional after-work drink with colleagues, he wasn't too interested in drinking alcohol. While his health history did include a diagnosis of chronic ulcerative colitis (an inflammation of the inner lining of his colon and rectum), that condition had been inactive for years.

His itching persisted for weeks, and anti-itch lotions weren't helping. He also noticed that he felt more fatigue than usual, but he shrugged it off as stress-related.

It wasn't until his company's annual blood drive that Ben received his first indication of trouble. The nurse who tested his blood told him that his "enzymes were elevated" and that he would not be permitted to donate blood that day. She reassured him, saying that a long list of harmless factors could raise enzyme levels, including extra workouts or a few drinks the night before the test. After diagnostic tests were performed, however, Ben learned that he had a disease known as primary sclerosing cholangitis, or PSC.

PSC: AN UNCOMMON DISEASE

It is a rare disorder, but PSC is easier to visualize than some liver diseases are. The liver, you will remember, excretes bile (the liquid that helps break down fat in our food) into the bile ducts, tiny tubes found

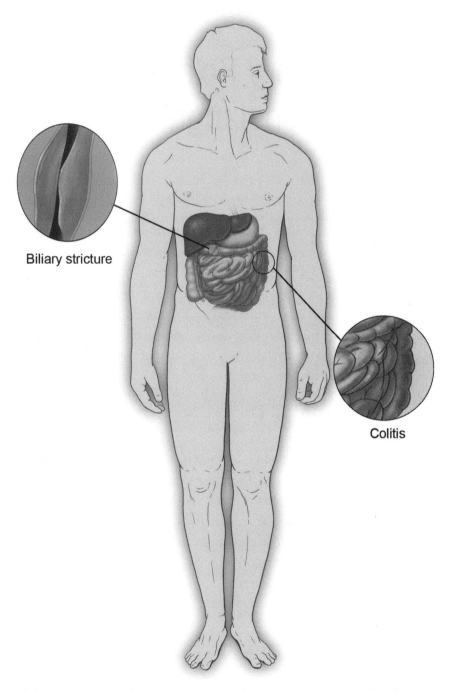

Biliary stricture

Colitis

Primary sclerosing cholangitis (PSC) causes inflammation and scarring of bile ducts both inside and outside the liver (biliary strictures). Frequently, people with PSC also have inflammatory bowel disease, more commonly referred to as colitis.

both inside the liver (intrahepatic ducts) and outside (extrahepatic). These ducts form an intricate network resembling filigreed jewelry or the veins on a leaf. Ultimately the bile ducts empty bile into the common bile duct, a bigger tube that leads into the intestine, where the bile helps digestion.

(A bit of health trivia: Bile is what gives stool its brown color; the color is that of the final product of bilirubin, the greenish-yellow pigment in bile.)

With primary sclerosing cholangitis (PSC), the walls of the bile ducts become inflamed (cholangitis), resulting in scarring, hardening, and over time a narrowing of the ducts. Because the ducts become narrower, PSC is known as a chronic cholestatic liver disease, or one in which bile cannot flow normally through the ducts. Both intrahepatic and extrahepatic ducts can be affected. At that stage, the bile accumulates in the liver, damaging the organ itself and developing into cirrhosis (hardening, or fibrosis, of the liver). Eventually, the liver will be too scarred and hardened to function, and it may fail.

PSC strikes infrequently, and it is difficult to detect because PSC patients display no symptoms in the early stages. Furthermore, most affected individuals show no symptoms when they're diagnosed or even until years later. Typically, the disease is discovered (as was the case for Ben) during a routine blood test. It is found more often in men than in women (about 70 percent of cases occur in men) and begins between the ages of 30 and 60. PSC progresses slowly; when symptoms do develop, they can include:

- Itching (pruritus), caused by too much bile in the bloodstream
- Fatigue
- Jaundice, leading to yellowing eyes and skin
- Pain in the upper right quadrant of the torso, caused by cholangitis, an inflammation or infection of the biliary system that may produce chills, fever, and pain
- As cirrhosis evolves, fluid swelling of the abdomen (ascites) and feet (edema), loss of appetite, and weight loss
- Muscle wasting

About 70 percent of PSC patients also need to be treated for ulcerative colitis, a disease in which the bowel becomes inflamed and colon ulcers develop. Many experts now believe that the connection between PSC and ulcerative colitis may be genetic.

WHAT CAUSES PSC?

No one knows the exact cause of PSC. Usually it is noticed when the patient's immune system changes or is stressed by a virus, bacteria, or an unrelated immunological disease. Genetics, too, are likely to play a role.

We *are* able to pin down elevated levels of two key enzymes, known as AP (alkaline phosphatase) and GGTP (gamma-glutamyl transpeptidase). When those heightened enzyme levels are detected, the physician will order a special diagnostic procedure with a complicated name: an endoscopic retrograde cholangiopancreatogram – for obvious reasons referred to simply as ERCP. (Occasionally, if an ERCP is not available or cannot be performed, MRCP – magnetic resonance cholangiopancreatography –may be employed instead.)

For an ERCP (during which the patient is sedated), a small lighted tube, or endoscope, is inserted into the mouth and threaded through the small intestine until it reaches a tiny intestinal opening called the *ampulla of Vater*, which leads to the extrahepatic bile ducts. A thinner tube is inserted into the ducts, creating access for a contrast dye that will highlight the ducts on an x-ray, enabling doctors to see them and determine whether they are damaged.

If the bile ducts are narrowed and irregular, a diagnosis of PSC is confirmed. In some cases narrowed bile ducts can be dilated or a stent (a small tube) can be inserted to keep a duct open. After these procedures, patients feel much better as bile begins to flow more freely. Nonetheless, new narrowings can still develop.

In some hospitals an MRCP may be performed. This is an MRI that looks at the biliary tree. However, the MRCP does not allow for dilation or stenting. It simply produces a diagnostic picture.

PSC is not a predictable disease. Symptoms may persist at the same level, occur intermittently, or steadily progress. In some patients, it takes 15 to 20 years before the liver deteriorates to the point of failure and a transplant must be considered.

As the disease slowly progresses, a biopsy will show the extent of damage to the liver, but rarely is biopsy used to make the initial diagnosis. PSC follows a "staging system" that gives insight into the patient's longer-term prognosis, with Stage 1 indicating early scarring and narrowing of the bile ducts, and Stage 4 carrying a diagnosis of cirrhosis.

GREAT TREATMENTS, BUT NO CURE

While PSC is an incurable disease, its symptoms can be treated effectively and its progression may be slowed. Certainly patients should sample the range of available anti-itch medications on the market, including prescription meds such as cholestyramine (Questran), which binds up bile salts in the intestine and allows them to be eliminated with stool, thereby reducing their accumulation in the liver and skin.

Patients can supplement their diets with vitamins A, D, and K – commonly deficient in PSC patients – if necessary.

More serious complications of PSC are osteoporosis and osteomalacia (bone-calcium deficiency). Patients are advised to increase their intake of calcium with vitamin D to boost absorption and to consider bone-density medications if these conditions are noted on a bone-density scan.

Gallstones, too, are frequently seen in PSC patients and can be treated as they are in patients who do not have PSC.

Two possible malignancies are linked to PSC. One is cholangiocarcinoma, or cancer of the bile ducts, and the second is colon cancer. PSC patients have a 10 percent to 15 percent lifetime chance of developing cancer in the bile ducts, most often when they have inflammatory bowel disease or cirrhosis. With a higher risk of colon cancer as well (especially patients with both PSC and ulcerative colitis), PSC patients are strongly advised to have annual colonoscopies.

When infections occur in the bile ducts, they should be treated with antibiotics. Restricted salt intake as well as use of diuretics can help reduce swelling of the abdomen and feet, once PSC becomes cirrhosis.

One of the most successful treatments for PSC is balloon dilation, or stenting, a procedure used to "open up" narrowed bile ducts; in fact, success rates of up to 85 percent have been reported with the initial dilation. In those procedures, the physician places a small balloon-tipped tube into the constricted duct; once it is in place the balloon is inflated to open up the duct and permit bile flow. Stents, or plastic tubes, often are inserted into the ducts to keep them open. In spite of this, renarrowing occurs in up to half of those patients, so the procedure usually must be repeated and the stents need to be changed.

Only one drug, ursodeoxycholic acid (marketed as Ursodiol and Actigall), is often used in PSC patients. However, it has not been definitively shown to improve survival or to delay the need for transplantation.

The ultimate concern connected with PSC is the possibility of liver failure, and the only option at that point is a liver transplant. Fortunately, liver transplantation has advanced to the point where it is a proven mainstream treatment for severe, chronic liver disease. The survival rate for liver-transplant patients now is well over the 90 percent mark, and those patients can expect a high quality of life after their recovery. Patients like Ben, whose symptoms probably can be managed for years with medications and supplements, can have every expectation of maintaining their normal life expectancies. ◆

A powerhouse performance: The liver is responsible for more than 500 processes that keep our bodies working efficiently. No other organ performs so many complex and vital functions for the body. The liver helps to digest food, manufactures proteins, stores many vital nutrients, and disposes of toxins. Without its help, our blood would be clogged with fats, glucose, and amino acids, and our bodies would have no defense against infections, no way to eliminate the drugs and toxins we consume, and no mechanism for processing digested food from the intestine.

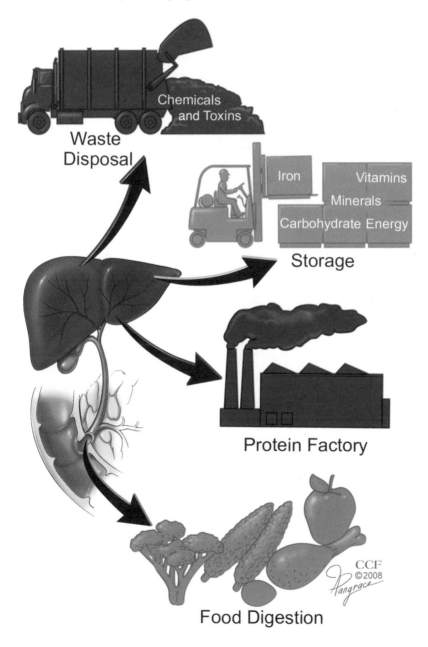

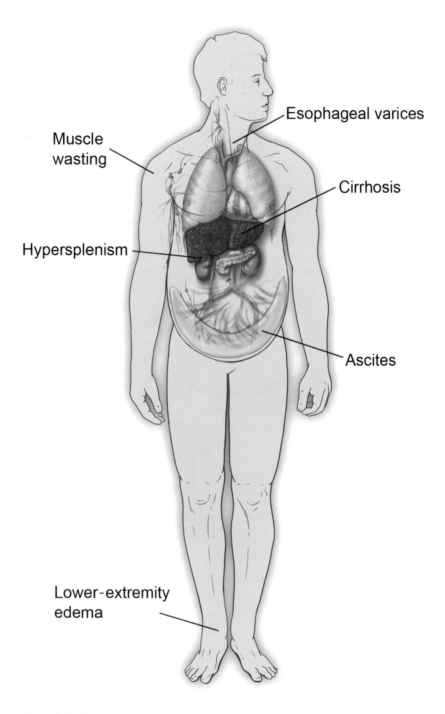

Esophageal varices

Muscle wasting

Cirrhosis

Hypersplenism

Ascites

Lower-extremity edema

Cirrhosis is characterized by a number of physical manifestations. A damaged liver causes many problems outside the liver itself.

Like Wilson disease (see page 64), hereditary hemochromatosis is an inherited condition involving a mineral overload in the blood. In this case the culprit is iron; in the case of Wilson disease, it is copper.

TIPSS: *A transjugular intra-hepatic portosystemic shunt. Generally used to control refractory variceal bleeding or refractory ascites, the stent (pictured in red) "shunts" the blood from the veins below the liver to those above, reducing portal pressures.*

Hepatitis C Infection: A Systemic Disease

Many extrahepatic syndromes can complicate hepatitis C virus (HCV) infection. Some are strongly linked to HCV, others are less strongly linked, and yet others are due to interferon treatment for HCV.

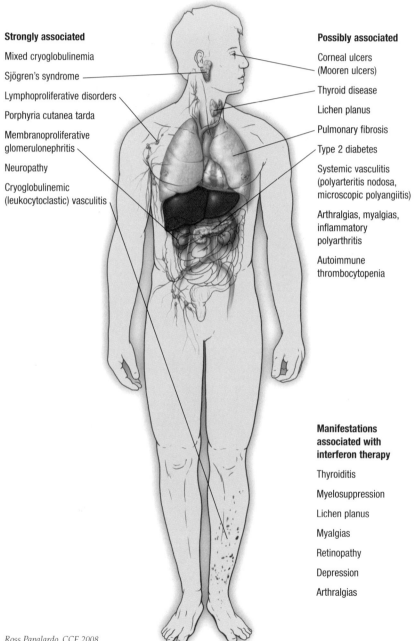

Strongly associated

Mixed cryoglobulinemia

Sjögren's syndrome

Lymphoproliferative disorders

Porphyria cutanea tarda

Membranoproliferative glomerulonephritis

Neuropathy

Cryoglobulinemic (leukocytoclastic) vasculitis

Possibly associated

Corneal ulcers (Mooren ulcers)

Thyroid disease

Lichen planus

Pulmonary fibrosis

Type 2 diabetes

Systemic vasculitis (polyarteritis nodosa, microscopic polyangiitis)

Arthralgias, myalgias, inflammatory polyarthritis

Autoimmune thrombocytopenia

Manifestations associated with interferon therapy

Thyroiditis

Myelosuppression

Lichen planus

Myalgias

Retinopathy

Depression

Arthralgias

Ross Papalardo, CCF 2008

Chapter 10

Liver Masses

For 66 years, Jeannette had been one of the lucky ones. Unlike so many of her friends, she didn't suffer the pains of arthritis. Her vision was still good, and unless the sidewalks were covered with snow, she walked two miles a day. Even in bad weather, she kept herself in good condition with an exercise video. Jeannette was a firm believer in the saying "When you rest, you rust."

So, as a person who was conscientious and informed about her health, Jeannette was concerned when she began feeling an achy tenderness in the upper right quadrant of her abdomen. She knew that discomfort in that spot could mean a liver problem. Jeannette sometimes enjoyed a glass of wine with dinner, but she hadn't smoked cigarettes since her college years. She couldn't think of anything in her lifestyle that would put her at risk for liver disease, but she remembered that almost all of her aunts and uncles had died from one type of cancer or another.

Jeannette wasted no time in making an appointment to see her doctor. Knowing that this patient took good care of herself, the doctor scheduled a CT scan to see whether any physical abnormalities on the liver would be apparent. It was a good choice of tests: A cyst was immediately visible, and by all appearances, the cyst was benign.

DIRECT ROUTE TO TUMORS

It is not unusual to hear that someone was diagnosed with a liver tumor (mass), and it is easy to understand why: The liver is like the freeway from the digestive system. Everything we ingest is processed by the liver – food, drinks, cigarette smoke, auto-exhaust fumes – so the liver, like the lungs, is an organ that carries a major risk of damage caused by materials we bring into our bodies. When serious damage (cancer, for example) occurs in a different part of the body, the liver's two blood suppliers, the portal vein and the hepatic artery, can bring cancerous tumor cells from those other organs and deposit them in the liver. This is how cancer from the digestive system and other organs metastasizes to the liver.

Another reason that liver tumors seem so common nowadays is the improved radiological equipment in hospitals; these machines are much better at detecting the tumors than the equipment used even a decade ago. Imaging techniques today enable doctors to identify benign masses on the liver as well as cancerous tumors, often by accident when they are investigating an unrelated condition or symptom.

Virtually every liver mass can be labeled as either a benign tumor or a malignant (cancerous) tumor. The only way to distinguish between the two is to perform a liver biopsy. Naturally, the hope is always that the mass is benign, in which case the tumor will not spread to other organs.

BENIGN TUMORS

While benign liver tumors occur in many forms, five types are far more common than the others: hemangiomas, hepatic adenomas, focal nodular hyperplasia, solitary liver cysts, and nodular regenerative hyperplasia – long names to identify liver masses that carry their own unique characteristics, symptoms, and treatments.

Hemangiomas

As their name implies, hemangiomas are filled with *heme*, or blood. In fact, they closely resemble the harmless red spots known as senile hemangiomas, which people discover on their chests and abdomens as they get older.

The most common type of benign liver tumor, hemangiomas are estimated to occur in up to 20 percent of the population; about one-tenth of those individuals – more women than men – will have more than one. Frequently, hemangiomas also are discovered in the brain, lungs, or skin. They can occur at any age.

Hemangiomas almost always remain small, and because they usually cause no symptoms, most people with these masses don't even realize they are there. Occasionally, the hemangioma will grow larger than a few centimeters, and this can cause pain in the upper right quadrant of the abdomen. If the hemangioma continues to expand, bleeding can occur within the tumor, forming blood clots within the tumor itself and causing pain in some cases.

It is rare for the hemangioma to bleed into the abdominal cavity, but it does happen – an extremely serious and painful event that calls for emergency surgery.

A hemangioma usually is discovered during a sonogram or CT scan given for an unrelated disorder. If the mass is larger than 2.5 centimeters, a tagged red blood cell (RBC) scan may be ordered – a test that "dyes" the blood with a radioactive metallic element called a tracer. The RBC scan is a rather lengthy test; it takes about two hours for the tracer to accumulate in the hemangioma before the diagnosis is confirmed.

If the hemangioma is greatly enlarged (more than 10 to 15 centimeters) or causes pain, surgical removal may be required. Otherwise, hemangiomas generally are left alone and should not undergo needle biopsy.

Hepatic Adenoma

Much less common than hemangiomas are hepatic adenomas, benign tumors usually found in women of childbearing age who have taken birth-control pills for at least five years or who have had several pregnancies. The link to estrogen is an obvious assumption.

The good news is that hepatic adenomas have become even more rare in recent decades as the amount of estrogen in birth-control pills has decreased.

About half of all hepatic adenoma patients complain of pain in the right upper quadrant of their abdomens, while many others detect no symptoms at all until the tumor ruptures, a serious and painful emergency requiring immediate surgery. For others, the tumor often is found during routine physical exams or when diagnostic studies are made for an unrelated disorder. CT scans and MRIs can help to locate the tumor, while a liver biopsy can confirm the diagnosis.

Although hepatic adenomas are benign, occasionally they lead to liver cancer, so treatment usually is indicated. The least invasive form of treatment is to stop the use of any prescriptions that contain estrogen. Often this approach is successful. If the tumor persists, surgery usually is the next step.

Doctors advise prospective mothers to defer pregnancy until the adenoma has been successfully treated because the mother's hormone fluctuations may cause the tumor to grow and rupture. Once the hepatic adenoma is gone, however, it is safe to go ahead with a pregnancy.

Focal Nodular Hyperplasia (FNH)

Another benign tumor more common to women is focal nodular hyperplasia (FNH), a mass of liver cells that multiply around a malformed hepatic artery. Most women experience no symptoms unless the tumor is greatly enlarged; at that point the patient may notice abdominal pain or a mass.

FNH is less worrisome than some other benign tumors because it rarely ruptures and never progresses to liver cancer. Typically, the tumor is discovered during a scan for an unrelated problem. The only treatment is to discontinue estrogen-containing medications because hormone imbalance, while not a proven cause of FNH, is thought to contribute to the tumor's growth. If the FNH is causing discomfort, the doctor might recommend surgical removal.

Liver Cysts

Like other kinds of cysts, a simple liver cyst is a sac that contains fluid. A common occurrence, it is sometimes found on the liver at birth, and usually appears in the liver's right lobe. And, like most benign liver tumors, solitary liver cysts are found more often in women than in men.

Usually, these cysts cause no symptoms and are detected during exams for other conditions. They can cause pain if they grow to more than 5 centimeters, and very occasionally they will bleed or become infected. In such instances, symptoms do appear – pain, fever, or elevated liver enzymes. Those cysts are likely to be treated with ablation therapy – a procedure in which alcohol or doxycycline (an antibiotic) is injected into the cyst, causing it to shrink and self-destruct, thereby ending the symptoms. If the cyst returns, it can be removed with surgery. Unless the cyst causes symptoms, no treatment is prescribed.

Nodular Regenerative Hyperplasia (NRH)

Possibly the most bizarre of the benign liver tumors, nodular regenerative hyperplasia (NRH) is a condition in which normal liver cells are replaced by nodules of continually regenerating liver cells. Usually it is found in individuals over the age of 50, and it is associated with a wide variety of conditions that don't involve the liver, including rheumatoid arthritis, some chemotherapies, amyloidosis (a disease where the protein amyloid is deposited in a number of organs), bone marrow or liver transplantation, and exposure to toxic substances.

Although NRH is believed to be a benign condition, liver cancer has developed in NRH patients. Rather than generating its own symptoms, NRH often is discovered when doctors are studying symptoms of its associated conditions. If left untreated, it could progress to affect the entire liver, in a fashion resembling the scarring caused by cirrhosis, and it has even resulted in liver failure.

Diagnosis is difficult. NRH usually will not show up on scans, and even a liver biopsy can miss the affected area. The only definitive way to diagnosis NRH is by a laparoscopic or a more substantial surgical biopsy of the liver. If the NRH progresses to portal hypertension, or if it causes cirrhosis-like scarring of too much liver tissue, then a liver transplant might be one of few options.

HEPATOCELLULAR CARCINOMA (HCC): LIVER CANCER

Although it is common for tumors that originate in other parts of the body to metastasize to the liver, a primary malignant liver tumor begins in the liver itself. The most common type of liver cancer is hepatocellular carcinoma, often called hepatoma or HCC – one of the most common cancers we know.

Up to 1 million new HCC cases are reported in the world each year, or about 6 percent of all cancers worldwide. It is the fifth most common cancer in men and the ninth most common in women, though in the United States it accounts for only about 2 percent of all cancers. Still, its numbers in this country are growing each year, possibly connected to the increase in cases of chronic hepatitis C.

Interestingly, HCC behaves differently in different countries: In Asia and Africa, where it is a more common cancer, HCC strikes at an early age and appears quite suddenly. In the United States, however,

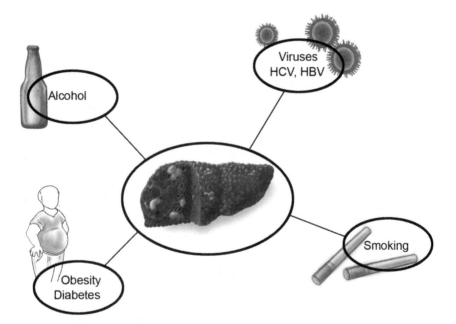

Hepatocellular carcinoma (HCC) is the most common form of liver cancer. Significant risk factors include a history of smoking and excessive alcohol consumption, and conditions such as obesity, diabetes, and hepatitis B and C.

it is seen most often in mature adults and grows very gradually. This is because of the link to hepatitis B and C. Hepatitis B is much more common in Asia and Africa and is usually acquired at birth or a very early age as opposed to hepatitis C, which is more common in the United States and acquired at a later age.

HCC's Causes and Connections

In an organ as busy as the liver, which filters every fume, liquid, and morsel of food that enters the body, cancer probably is triggered by many factors. The clearest association we know is with cirrhosis, but it is also possible that lifestyle choices (particularly alcohol abuse), viruses, chemical exposure, genetics, hormones, aging, and even nutrition also influence the onset of HCC.

The connection between cirrhosis and liver cancer could not be clearer. Cirrhosis is found in up to 90 percent of HCC patients. Conversely, more than a quarter of cirrhosis patients also had undiagnosed HCC, according to autopsy studies.

Patients with chronic hepatitis B (HBV) or hepatitis C (HCV) also have a high risk of developing liver cancer: HBV has been shown to be a leading cause of HCC, accounting for up to 75 percent of all liver cancers. Even when cirrhosis is not diagnosed, HCC can be found in HBV patients, possibly because of a gene that can make an individual more vulnerable to contracting HCC. HBV is a DNA virus, and it is possible that gene mutations occur in HBV patients that help usher in HCC.

If the patient carries both HBV and HCV, chances are even higher that he or she will contract liver cancer, a development that is greatly exacerbated if the patient is a heavy alcohol drinker. In fact, in chronic hepatitis B and C patients who drink to excess, HCC appears an average of 10 years earlier than it does in those who do not drink alcohol. (Usually, it takes 20 to 30 years before HCC manifests in an HBV patient.) Clearly, anyone diagnosed with HBV is advised to avoid alcohol, thereby possibly postponing the onset of cancer.

Hepatitis C, too, is strongly linked to liver cancer. Unlike patients with hepatitis B, cirrhosis exists in virtually all HCC patients whose cancer derives from chronic hepatitis C.

Hemochromatosis, a disease of "iron overload," will not in itself cause HCC, but once cirrhosis has developed, the patient's risk of contracting HCC jumps to 200 times that of the general population. For hemochromatosis patients whose livers are not yet cirrhotic, phlebotomy can help to head off HCC. While other liver diseases (including nonalcoholic fatty liver disease, autoimmune hepatitis, and primary biliary cirrhosis) also carry the potential of progressing to cirrhosis and, eventually, to HCC, the correlation between HCC and hepatitis B, hepatitis C, and hemochromatosis is far stronger.

Not surprisingly, one's lifestyle can be a major contributing factor to HCC. The point is made many times in this book that alcohol is toxic to the liver; while alcohol itself does not cause HCC, it does cause cirrhosis and other liver damage, and renders the liver much more vulnerable to cancer. About 15 percent of patients with alcoholic cirrhosis, in fact, will eventually develop HCC. And while the direct effects of tobacco on the liver are not yet known, some studies do show a link between smoking and HCC in patients with liver disorders.

Some readers will be surprised to find a connection between HCC and aflatoxin, a byproduct of aspergillus flavus (in simple terms, a mold) that happens to be toxic to the liver. Aflatoxin contamination can occur in foods stored in hot, humid places for extended periods. It is possible that aflatoxin acts as a cocarcinogen – a substance that can lead to cancer development when combined with other cancer-causing agents. While it is rare in the United States, aflatoxin contamination is not uncommon in stored corn, rice, peanuts, and soybeans in certain Asian and African regions.

Even diabetes may put people at increased risk of developing liver cancer. Many extensive studies have shown that patients with diabetes and obesity are at an increased risk for developing a number of different types of cancer, including hepatocellular carcinoma. There might also be a link between HCC and patients with NASH (nonalcoholic steatohepatitis), because many of those individuals have diabetes, hyperinsulinemia, or both.

Since men develop HCC two to four times as often as women do, gender is viewed as a factor, possibly because of increased cases of alcoholic cirrhosis and viral hepatitis in men. Ethnicity, too, is a factor: Asians, Hispanics, Native Americans, and African Americans all contract HCC more often than Caucasians do. This may be due to such lifestyle differences as varying rates of alcohol consumption, tobacco use, diabetes, and hepatitis B and C among different ethnic groups. More likely this difference is due to the genetic differences in disease susceptibility (susceptible genes).

Finally, although aging does not cause cancer, the cumulative effect of gene damage from all the above causes makes HCC in this country a disease of mature adults. It is rarely seen in men or women younger than 40 years of age.

Common Contributors to HCC	Strength of Association (+ to +++)
Alcohol	+
Smoking	+
Diabetes	+
Obesity	+
Viral Hepatitis B	++
Viral Hepatitis C	++
Cirrhosis	+++

SYMPTOMS AND DIAGNOSIS OF HCC

As we've noted, geography matters in discussing malignant liver tumors. In the United States, HCC often is diagnosed early, when the tumor is tiny – but the diagnosis often results from regular cirrhosis monitoring rather than the appearance of symptoms of the cancer itself. We also see cases, however, in which sudden symptoms appear, such as dramatic weight loss, fatigue, abdominal pain, or mild jaundice. There may also be clear signs of decompensated cirrhosis, such as ascites (accumulation of fluid in the abdomen).

About 5 percent of HCC patients experience paraneoplastic syndrome, or HCC-related symptoms that show up in other parts of the body. Two examples are hypoglycemia (a low glucose level) and hypercholesterolemia (a high cholesterol level). Elevated calcium levels and red blood cell count, watery diarrhea, and high blood pressure are other symptoms seen with this syndrome.

As with most liver diseases, diagnosing HCC usually entails a series of tests, including blood work, imaging studies, and possibly a liver biopsy. Only one blood test is commonly used to assist in the detection of HCC: the alpha-fetoprotein, or AFP. Known as a "tumor marker" because it can detect HCC, an AFP can show the presence of cancer if the blood level is above 400 nanograms per milliliter (ng/ml). HCC also is indicated if the level is still relatively low but has escalated dramatically within a few months. Otherwise, a reading of under 400 ng/ml can point to other possible conditions.

Typically, a sonogram, CT scan, or MRI is ordered also. When the physician is considering surgery, a hepatic angiography might also be performed. This is an invasive test that involves placing a catheter in the hepatic artery and injecting a dye into the vessels that carry blood to the tumor.

When a tumor has been detected but not diagnosed, doctors sometimes will order a liver biopsy – but the test is not without risks. Liver tumors are overly vascular (full of veins), so performing a needle biopsy carries a risk of bleeding.

HCC PATIENTS AND THE FUTURE

As with most cancers, early detection and diagnosis of HCC is key to the patient's long-term survival. This involves frequent screening of patients who are at risk of developing HCC, including any individual with cirrhosis and those with chronic hepatitis B. It is estimated that with a sonogram and an AFP blood test performed at least every six months, between 25 and 65 percent of tumors measuring two centimeters or smaller can be detected.

When a liver tumor smaller than five to seven centimeters has been found and diagnosed, chances are good that it can be successfully removed with surgery. Tumors larger than seven centimeters probably cannot be removed because by the time they reach that size, it is likely that the cancer has metastasized to other organs and more aggressive therapies are needed.

When a liver tumor smaller than five to seven centimeters has been found and diagnosed, chances are good that it can be successfully removed with surgery.

A range of treatment options is available to HCC patients: surgical resection, liver transplants, alcohol injections, and more. Combining several treatments often can maximize one's chances of survival, though a number of factors – including the number and size of tumors, and the presence and status of other liver diseases – will help determine the outcome.

In many instances, surgical resection (removal of the tumor by surgery) is the best option, because if cirrhosis has not developed, up to 60 percent of a patient's liver can be removed and it will still regenerate, or grow back to its normal size. If cirrhosis is absent, resection is most successful in otherwise healthy patients who present only one tumor less than five centimeters in size. Of those patients who undergo surgical resection, about half are still alive five years later.

However, only about 5 percent of HCC patients are good candidates for surgical resection. For the others, an increasingly successful choice is liver transplantation, a good option for HCC patients who have developed cirrhosis. For these patients, the five-year survival rate is 75 percent, though the waiting period can be an obstacle. In those instances, a living-donor transplantation – a procedure in which part of a liver is donated by a compatible donor and transplanted into the HCC patient – can be a lifesaver.

Because liver tumors grow so gradually and imperceptibly, many become inoperable by the time they are diagnosed. For those patients, one option is a percutaneous alcohol injection (PEI), in which alcohol is injected by needle into the tumor – a procedure that "kills" up to 90 percent of small tumors (of less than five centimeters) in patients who have fewer than three liver tumors and who have not developed advanced cirrhosis.

For individuals with a larger tumor, doctors may try tumor embolization and chemoembolization. They would selectively introduce chemotherapy drugs into a branch of the hepatic artery supplying the HCC. Gelfoam gelatin sponges containing the drugs often are used to offer the best chance of killing the cancer cells.

Another popular treatment for liver tumors is radiofrequency ablation (RFA), which uses heat caused by electrical energy to kill the cancerous tissue. During the procedure, a special probe is inserted into the tumor. When it is positioned correctly, several electrodes protruding from the tip of the probe send a predetermined amount of radiofrequency, or "heat energy," into the tissue. Tiny thermometers in the device measure the heat until the cancerous tissue is dead. It is a relatively quick procedure, usually lasting less than 15 minutes, and is done with appropriate anesthesia.

Several newer treatments are still under study. One systemic chemotherapeutic agent known as sorafenib is showing some effectiveness in delaying growth of nonresectable HCC. Hormonal therapy, branching out from the premise that hormones can influence the growth of tumors, shows promise. Interferons, the "burning" of tumor cells, gene therapy, cryosurgery (the freezing of cancerous tumor cells), and anti-angiogenesis (which prevents the formation new blood vessels needed by the tumor), are all being studied and may lead to more successful HCC treatments in the future.

WHEN A TUMOR ISN'T A LIVER CANCER

Because liver tumors share so many symptoms with other illnesses, a primary liver cancer can closely resemble other afflictions.

Three of those disorders are based in the liver. The most serious is a metastatic liver tumor, a cancer that began in some other organ and spread to the liver. Metastatic liver tumors, which often begin in the colon, kidney, uterus, lungs, stomach, gallbladder, breast, esophagus, or pancreas, are much more common than primary liver cancers.

Another liver condition that can be mistaken for primary liver cancer is a pseudotumor. Made of regenerating cirrhosis nodules, the pseudotumor nodules often cluster and may give the appearance of a tumor mass.

Also capable of fooling imaging equipment is a "focal fatty infiltration" of the liver, or fat deposits clumped together to give the appearance of a tumor. Obesity, alcoholic liver disease, and diabetes are all potential causes; when the underlying condition is corrected, the fat deposits may disappear.

The alpha-fetoprotein (AFP) blood test, too, can mislead patients and doctors. Earlier in this chapter, this test was presented as a tumor marker – a test that can detect but not diagnose HCC with elevated blood levels. However, a higher-than-normal AFP result also could indicate pregnancy, cystic fibrosis, gastric cancer, pancreatic cancer, metastatic liver cancer (as opposed to HCC, in which the liver is the primary organ where the cancer originated), or cirrhosis.

With all liver disorders – but especially when a cancerous tumor is suspected – patients should remember that making premature assumptions can be hazardous to one's health! Clearly, a series of diagnostic procedures, rather than conclusions drawn from one blood test, represents the best path to a positive long-term prognosis.

And as with most cancers, *early detection* is key to the patient's long-term survival. It is important to understand that many liver-related symptoms – jaundice, unexplained weight loss, diminished appetite, and abdominal pain, among others – may signal HCC or a precancerous condition.

It is no longer true that a diagnosis of liver cancer means that the patient is doomed; HCC, if detected early, now is considered one of the "curable cancers." But to ensure a successful outcome, it must be detected and treated *early*. ◆

LIVER CANCER *CAN* BE PREVENTED

Liver cancer is not only curable, it is often preventable. Lifestyle choices often contribute to the likelihood that an individual will contract HCC. As you can see from the following list, most of the strategies for avoiding liver cancer merely involve not putting yourself at risk.

- **Never, ever smoke.** Did you really need another reason to quit smoking tobacco?

- **Limit your drinking.** Alcohol damages the liver. If your liver is healthy, alcohol abuse can cause cirrhosis. If you already have a liver disorder, too much alcohol will accelerate the disease.

- **Exercise and maintain a healthy weight.** Obesity and insulin resistance cause NAFLD (fatty liver disease) and contribute to other liver disorders. Keep your liver healthy with a heart-healthy diet and regular exercise.

- **Avoid exposure to hepatitis B (HBV) and hepatitis C (HCV).** People who engage in unprotected sex or share IV needles (including those used in giving tattoos), or who live with an HBV or HCV patient, are at risk for those diseases. Never share needles or have unprotected sex.

- **If you are at risk for hepatitis B, take the HBV vaccination.** This includes families of HBV patients; the vaccine will protect you from contracting the disease. Currently, it is recommended that all infants in the U.S. receive the hepatitis B vaccine series.

- **Never take anabolic steroids.** These are the steroids that have made headlines when professional athletes have taken them. Anabolic steroids may cause cancer.

- **Learn about aflatoxins.** Aflatoxins are cancer-causing toxins produced by a mold. They grow on the skins of corn, peanuts, rice, potatoes, and other such foods. The United States tests for aflatoxins, but it is a good idea to buy foods grown in your own region, rather than those transported from hot, humid locales where molds can grow on stored food.

Chapter 11

Cirrhosis and Its Complications

Andrew, in his late 50s, considered himself a successful guy. Every aspect of his life, in fact, was in great shape: Owner of an auto body shop, Andrew was happily married to his high school sweetheart, his three children had graduated from college and were making their way in the world, and he was financially secure. He had good friends and a time-share in South Carolina, and he was healthy. Or so he thought.

Andrew showed restraint at lunch – he never had more than one beer. He did stop after work for a bourbon or two with his buddies, just until the rush-hour crowd diminished. It was a comfortable way to end the day. It wouldn't occur to him to "tie one on" after work – the truth was, he loved going home. Sometimes he drank a glass of wine with dinner, but it wasn't a nightly ritual.

When Andrew began feeling vague symptoms, he ignored them. After all, he didn't eat red meat, he exercised four days a week, and he made sure that his diet included plenty of fiber. Andrew considered himself to be a health-aware sort of person, and his symptoms – fatigue, weight loss, occasional nausea – easily could be explained as flu symptoms. Why would he look for a serious disorder?

When he had to add an ache in his upper right abdomen to the list of his other symptoms, his wife finally put her foot down. It was time to see a doctor. No one was more surprised than Andrew when, after a battery of tests, the diagnosis was confirmed: Incredibly, Andrew had cirrhosis of the liver! Because he restricted his alcohol intake to about four drinks a day, he wasn't about to believe the diagnosis without a second opinion.

The diagnosis held true. Tests for liver diseases linked to cirrhosis (such as chronic hepatitis B and C, nonalcoholic steatohepatitis, PBC, PSC, autoimmune hepatitis, and Wilson disease) ruled out those disorders as possible causes. Andrew's cirrhosis was determined to be caused by alcoholic liver disease, which can develop in men who consume as little as four drinks per day.

SCARRING AND THE LIVER

With most injuries a scar is good news, indicating that repair and healing have begun. It is ironic, therefore, that in the case of cirrhosis, advanced scarring means that the liver is beyond repair. It is perhaps the most serious consequence of liver diseases – although, with the advances of modern medicine, cirrhosis isn't always the signal of doom that it once was.

As cirrhosis develops, scarred tissue replaces the healthy liver. Blood can no longer flow freely through the liver, and as the organ becomes hard and lumpy, its function deteriorates. This condition kills about 27,000 people each year, making it the 10th leading cause of death for men and the 12th for women in the United States.

We've known about cirrhosis and its effects for many centuries. It is believed that back in the 4th century B.C. Hippocrates said, "In cases of jaundice it is a bad sign when the liver becomes hard." In 18th-century England, cirrhosis was known as "gin liver" – a disease that developed when a surplus of corn crops brought an abundance of gin. Before 1820, French medical researcher René Laennec named the disease *cirrhose*, deriving the term from the Greek word *kirrhos*, meaning "tawny" – the orange-tan color of cirrhotic livers.

CAUSES OF CIRRHOSIS

The list of diseases and other causes that trigger cirrhosis is long and diverse, but you'll note that most of the causes are some form of liver disease:

- **Alcoholic liver disease.** This is, of course, the popular image of cirrhosis – a disease that strikes heavy drinkers. It usually takes a decade or longer of heavy drinking before alcoholic cirrhosis develops, but the amount of liquor that must be consumed is an individual thing. For men, three to four drinks a day can bring the initial scarring; for women, two to three. Alcohol is a toxin that directly damages the liver and prevents normal metabolism of protein, fats, and carbohydrates.

- **Chronic hepatitis C.** As the hepatitis C virus causes inflammation in the liver over several decades, the scarring damage happens very gradually, but it can be permanent.

- **Chronic hepatitis B and D.** Worldwide, the hepatitis B virus might be the most prevalent cause of cirrhosis, but this virus is less common in the United States; like hepatitis C, it works its damage on the liver for several decades before cirrhosis sets in. Hepatitis D, too, attacks the liver, but only in patients already suffering from hepatitis B; the co-infection accelerates the cirrhosis.

- **Nonalcoholic steatohepatitis.** In NASH, often linked to diabetes, obesity, coronary artery disease, and other components of the metabolic syndrome, the cirrhosis is brought on by fat and inflammation developing for years in the liver. The ill effects of NASH are similar to that of ALD, but without the influence of alcohol.

- **Primary biliary cirrhosis.** PBC patients may experience fatigue, pruritus (itching), and pigment changes to the skin, or they may notice no symptoms at all. Cirrhosis from PBC is more common in women than in men. The disease is confirmed with a liver biopsy.

- **Primary sclerosing cholangitis.** Symptoms leading to a PSC diagnosis can include pruritus, steatorrhea (excessively fatty stools), and fat-soluble vitamin deficiencies. PSC patients often have metabolic bone disease as well, and there is a strong correlation with inflammatory bowel disease (IBD).

- **Autoimmune hepatitis.** This disease, caused by immunologic damage to the liver (which inflames the liver and eventually brings on cirrhosis), is sometimes detected with elevations in liver enzymes and serum globulins. In cases of cirrhosis resulting from autoimmune hepatitis, the prognosis is very optimistic: The 10-year survival rate is more than 90 percent.

- **Hereditary hemochromatosis.** This disease of iron overload, with symptoms including skin hyperpigmentation, diabetes mellitus, and cardiomyopathy, is treated with phlebotomy to lower the body's iron levels.

- **Wilson disease** (an excess of copper in the liver), **cardiac cirrhosis** (caused by right-sided heart failure, leading to liver congestion and cirrhosis), **cystic fibrosis,** certain **drugs,** and certain **infections caused by parasites,** are less common causes of cirrhosis.

SYMPTOMS AND DIAGNOSIS OF CIRRHOSIS

In most instances, cirrhosis patients will first exhibit symptoms of the diseases that led to the development of the cirrhosis. It is the quintessential example of one disease "piggybacking" on or evolving into another.

In addition to those disease-specific symptoms, many other signs of cirrhosis can occur, either because of the scarring itself or because of other complications:

- Spider veins, spider angioma (a tiny artery with a network of red branches around it), or spider telangiectasia (elevated dark red blotches caused by chronically dilated groups of capillaries)

- Exaggerated speckled mottling of the palms of the hands known as palmar erythema

- Fingernail changes, including Muehrcke's nails (horizontal bands, usually seen in pairs, separated by normal nail-bed coloring), Terry's nails (in which two-thirds of the nail bed are white), and clubbing

- Certain finger deformities known as Dupuytren's contracture
- Breast growth in males, with sometimes tender, rubbery, or firm tissue behind the nipples, known as gynecomastia
- Impotence, infertility, and loss of sexual drive
- Change in liver size, either shrunken or enlarged
- Ascites, or accumulation of fluid in the abdomen
- Fetor hepatis, a distinctive, sweet, pungent odor on the breath
- Jaundice of the skin and eyes
- Weakness, fatigue, weight loss, and anorexia

Patients who have been diagnosed with a liver disease that can result in cirrhosis have in all likelihood been counseled regarding the possibility that cirrhosis could develop. They and their physicians will be alert for symptoms beyond those of their primary diseases.

Once cirrhosis is suspected, the most definitive test is a liver biopsy, though in many cases the biopsy is unnecessary if cirrhosis is indicated by the results of clinical, laboratory, and radiologic tests. A liver biopsy is invasive and carries recognized risks, so most physicians will avoid using it if there is increased risk of bleeding; they will rely instead on less invasive and more indirect signs and tests.

Lab indicators of cirrhosis include a low platelet count and perhaps moderately elevated aminotransferases (AST and ALT) with AST levels that are higher than those of the ALT. Alkaline phosphatase (AP) often will be slightly higher, as will the GGTP. As the cirrhosis progresses, the bilirubin may elevate and prothrombin time may increase, as will globulins, while the serum albumin level may fall. Because the liver plays a major role in blood coagulation, that process will be less efficient as the cirrhosis progresses, as indicated by the prolonged protime and low platelets.

The doctor also may order an ultrasound. Along with showing the altered size and nodular appearance that the liver takes on with advanced cirrhosis, the ultrasound also can screen for complications such as hepatocellular carcinoma (primary liver cancer) and portal hypertension. A CT scan of the abdomen and MRI of the liver and bile ducts may also be ordered.

Ascites (right) is an accumulation of fluid within the abdominal (peritoneal) cavity. It frequently appears in connection with cirrhosis.

Complications of cirrhosis and portal hypertension frequently include asterixis (below), an involuntary tremor of the wrist also known as "liver flap." This condition arises when the liver cannot properly filter the blood, enabling toxins to enter the brain.

Ascites

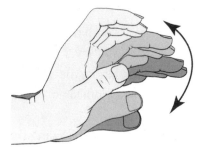

COMPLICATIONS OF CIRRHOSIS

As the scarring on the liver advances, complications may develop. One of the most common – and serious – is portal hypertension, or increased pressure within the portal vein (which carries blood from the digestive system to the liver), caused by the restriction of blood flow in the liver.

Portal hypertension carries its own set of symptoms, including black stools, vomiting blood, ascites, encephalopathy (confusion due to poor liver function and blood flow bypassing the liver), and a low white blood cell or platelet count. Medications such as propranolol to lower the blood pressure behind the liver and endoscopic therapy are treatment options for esophageal varices.

As a consequence of portal hypertension, the formation of varices, or large veins under the lining of the esophagus and stomach, is another complication. Varices develop as a way of bypassing the blockages to blood flow. These veins are fragile and pose a danger of bleeding, so they call for separate treatment. One method, known as TIPS shunting (see page 121), is usually performed only after an episode of bleeding from the varices. In this treatment, a small shunt is passed through the liver to relieve the pressure behind it. The other, more common, approach is to perform esophageal band ligation of the varices (placing rubber bands around the blood vessels) in the esophagus to block the flow of blood in these fragile vessels. The blood then finds an alternate route back to the heart through vessels not so prone to rupturing.

Other complications of cirrhosis – some of which can actually act as first signals to alert the patient and doctor that cirrhosis has begun – include:

- Jaundice, which appears because there is less processing of bilirubin, a greenish bile pigment
- Bruising and bleeding that occurs as coagulation becomes dysfunctional
- Itching (pruritus), a reaction to bile products in the skin

- Hepatic encephalopathy, caused when fewer toxins are cleared from the blood and instead circulate to the brain, resulting in forgetfulness, difficulty with concentration, and other mental symptoms

- Sensitivity to medications, the result of inefficient metabolism of drug ingredients

- Infections resulting from immune-system dysfunction

- Hepatocellular carcinoma, a primary liver cancer

- Scores of possible problems in other organs, in particular the kidneys, produced by insufficient processing of the blood

TREATMENT AND PROGNOSIS

Treating an irreversible condition such as cirrhosis of the liver is a complex and delicate process. Not only does cirrhosis follow on the heels of so many other diseases needing treatment, but as the section on complications shows, it also *causes* so many secondary conditions – all of which need treatment as well.

First, the patient should avoid any substance that can be harmful to the liver, including alcohol and excessive amounts of acetaminophen. A healthy diet that provides adequate calories and protein is recommended, and it may be necessary to restrict salt.

The patient should avoid any substance that can be harmful to the liver, including alcohol and excessive amounts of acetaminophen.

Beyond those general rules, treatment often is predicated on the disease that first caused the cirrhosis. Hepatitis-based cirrhosis calls for an appropriate treatment for the specific hepatitis, such as interferon therapy for viral hepatitis and corticosteroids in the case of autoimmune hepatitis. When Wilson disease, characterized by an accumulation of copper in the organs, causes the cirrhosis, chelation therapy to remove the copper is indicated.

When the complications overwhelm all prescribed treatments, the only recourse may be a liver transplant.

TREATING THE COMPLICATIONS OF CIRRHOSIS

Although cirrhosis itself is an irreversible condition, treating the *complications* of cirrhosis can prolong the patient's life and – perhaps more important – greatly improve its quality. With effective treatment of the complications listed below, a person with cirrhosis can live normally for many years.

- **Ascites, or fluid buildup in the abdomen.** The simplest and least invasive treatment for ascites is to restrict sodium intake and prescribe diuretics ("water pills") such as furosemide (Lasix) and spironolactone (Aldactone). If those steps don't control the ascites, then the physician may need to perform a paracentesis, or abdominal "tap" – a puncturing of the abdomen with a needle to draw off the fluid. If more treatment is needed, the doctor may recommend a TIPS, which is a stent (or tube) otherwise known as a transjugular intrahepatic portosystemic shunt. In this procedure, the TIPS will connect portal veins to adjacent blood vessels that are not affected by high blood pressure, thereby relieving the pressure of blood flowing through the diseased liver and lessening the fluid buildup.

- **Hepatic encephalopathy.** Caused by liver disease, this damage to the brain or nervous system presents such mental and physical symptoms as slowed reflexes, forgetfulness, sleepiness, and drastic changes in behavior. Hepatic encephalopathy is treated in several ways. The patient is asked to reduce his or her intake of animal protein, which in turn will reduce the production of ammonia. Lactulose, a type of synthetic sugar, often is given to increase alertness, and antibiotics such as Flagyl (metronidazole), neomycin, and rifaximin are prescribed to help stem the production of ammonia and other toxins.

- **Esophageal varices (dilated veins) and variceal bleeding.**
The doctor will consider prescribing a noncardioselective
beta-blocker – a medication that reduces the heart's work and
lowers blood pressure. Noncardioselective beta-blockers also
decrease the "blood pressure" behind the liver. The problem is
that when there is pressure behind the liver, blood cannot get
through the scarred liver. This leads to the formation of
esophageal varices that can eventually rupture. Another
treatment for esophageal varices is endoscopic band ligation
(described on page 119).

- **Malnutrition and wasting muscles.** These complications of
cirrhosis should be treated with a healthy diet, vitamin
replacement, and appropriate physical activity. The physician
can work with a nutritionist and an exercise physiologist to
determine the best diet and exercise plans for the patient.

- **Liver transplant.** This is not a complication, but a solution.
Liver transplantation is commonly performed when the liver is
seriously failing as a result of cirrhosis. Thanks to modern
surgical techniques and highly successful antirejection
medications, transplant surgery outcomes have greatly
improved. This option should be considered when the sum of
all the complications of cirrhosis threatens survival.

- **Medications.** Various medications can be prescribed for
patients in different stages of cirrhosis, depending on their liver
profiles and types of complications. (see Appendix C). ◆

Chapter 12

Pregnancy, Pediatrics, and the Liver

It took about a week for little Jonathan Whitman's parents to realize that their baby's behavior was unusual. Stu Whitman worked long hours managing a busy deli, so although he was an experienced dad with two children from a first marriage, most of the baby's care was up to Jonathan's mother, Teresa.

Jonathan's irritability came on suddenly, when he was about 6 weeks old, but Teresa thought he probably was reacting to his new formula. As a first-time mother, she didn't think his crankiness was out of the ordinary – after all, didn't all babies cry a lot? His stools became very light-colored, but Teresa shrugged that off as well, assuming that they had changed color with the new formula. She expected that Jonathan would adjust in a few days.

When Jonathan's dad noticed a yellowish tint to the baby's skin, however, they became alarmed and took him to their pediatrician the next morning. They were immediately referred to a liver specialist who was experienced in treating children, and after testing, the doctor's suspicions were confirmed: Jonathan was showing signs of biliary atresia; that is, his bile ducts had not fully developed, and the condition was preventing bile from draining out of his liver.

Because his parents hadn't recognized Jonathan's subtle symptoms right away, his condition had deteriorated rapidly. Doctors decided that the baby needed a liver transplant. Stu and Teresa thought a transplant was an extreme step to take with their baby, but the doctors convinced them that Jonathan needed the surgery in order to survive. They were able to perform the transplant before any permanent damage to Jonathan's growth and development occurred, and it was entirely successful: Three years later, Jonathan was playing as vigorously as any toddler – a strong, happy, perfectly healthy boy.

SPECIAL GROUPS, UNUSUAL CIRCUMSTANCES

Two special groups present unusual circumstances in connection with liver health: children and pregnant women. Certain disorders are more frequently seen in these groups than in the general adult population, and they sometimes display very special symptoms and signs. The treatments and prognoses, too, can be different for children and pregnant women. In this chapter, we highlight some of the more important features of these conditions.

PEDIATRIC LIVER DISEASE

Learning that a child has liver disease can be devastating news for parents, and certainly it is a serious matter, whatever the disorder. Today, fortunately, most pediatric liver diseases are fully treatable and not at all the disastrous illnesses they once were.

All parents should understand that jaundice is a common condition in newborns. Many babies develop jaundice in the first two or three days after their birth, and it generally disappears in about 10 days. If parents notice that their baby's jaundice has continued beyond that time, though, it is possible that causes other than the "normal" jaundice of the newly born are affecting the liver, and the baby should see a doctor immediately.

Inherited Pediatric Liver Diseases

A number of pediatric liver diseases, while quite manageable, are inherited. Parents whose babies are at risk for these diseases should be informed about the symptoms and consequences, and their children should be screened:

- **Ornithine transcarbamylase deficiency (OTC).** Produced by an abnormal gene that prevents newborns from processing excess ammonia in the system, OTC causes a newborn's ammonia levels to rise. The most effective treatment is an early liver transplant after careful evaluation.

- **Galactosemia.** An intolerance to sugars found in mother's and cow's milk causes one in 5,000 to 10,000 babies to develop this disease. Among the symptoms are lethargy, jaundice, and excessive sleepiness, with the baby not engaging or playing the way most babies do. If galactosemia is detected and diagnosed early, a switch to a galactose-free formula may be all the treatment that is needed.

- **Tyrosinemia.** Because tyrosinemia is so rare (just one in 100,000 infants is diagnosed in some regions), babies are not routinely screened for this disease, which causes toxins to accumulate in the liver. Evidence of the condition usually appears in the first several months of life. These babies are generally lethargic and jaundiced, display an enlarged abdomen, and appear to be seriously ill.

- **Biliary atresia.** This is the most common disease that leads to liver transplants in children, but it is eminently treatable. In biliary atresia, the bile ducts don't develop normally and bile cannot drain from the liver properly. When it appears in newborns, the infants may appear well for their first several weeks before developing a persistent jaundice. Irritability also may be present, as well as light-colored stools. Many children with biliary atresia undergo the surgical Kasai procedure, which helps the bile flow normally from the liver to the intestine, but about 80 percent of those patients eventually need a liver transplant. These transplant patients can expect an 80 percent to 90 percent chance of long-term survival – but without either the Kasai procedure or a transplant, infants may not survive, so early treatment is extremely important.

● **Alpha 1-antitrypsin (A1AT) deficiency.** This is an inherited disorder caused by an abnormal gene that controls the liver's production of a vital protein. This protein helps neutralize certain inflammatory enzymes in the body tissues. When the defective protein is produced, there can be damaging effects on the liver quite early in life, causing a picture of "hepatitis" in the newborn child. In fact, A1AT deficiency is the commonest cause of neonatal hepatitis. Sometimes the effects of the deficiency are delayed until later childhood or even adult life. The condition is diagnosed with a simple blood test (A1AT phenotype), which provides information on the genetic abnormality, and a liver biopsy, which shows the abnormal protein in the liver and any damage or scarring resulting from it. Like many other inherited liver diseases, it is effectively cured by a liver transplant.

Detecting Liver Disease in Children

As with adults, liver disease can be difficult to spot in children because the symptoms so often mimic those of less serious illnesses. The most important point for parents to remember is that many liver-related symptoms in children can be spotted in subtle behavior changes.

For instance, lethargy is a frequent clue; it can signal a metabolic abnormality or vitamin deficiency caused by a liver problem. Disorientation or confusion is another. Bleeding, the tendency to bruise easily, delayed growth, and simply acting "clingy" or too tired to play seem like subtle behaviors that all children experience from time to time, but they all can point to a liver-related diagnosis. Parents alerted to such problems need to observe their children closely and objectively to see whether any such abnormal patterns of behavior emerge.

Almost all pediatric liver diseases can be cured or managed effectively with early detection and treatment.

THE GENETIC PUZZLE

The gene for **alpha 1-antitrypsin** production resides on chromosome 14. This gene can mutate into several forms (M, S, Z). The form it takes will determine what type of A1AT the liver produces and how much deficiency occurs.

So what does this mean for the person affected?

- If you obtain an alpha 1-antitrypsin DNA test and you are shown to have phenotype MM, your genes/alleles in this area are considered "normal."

- If you are shown to have phenotype ZZ, you are *predisposed* to develop liver disease. It is not absolutely inevitable; some people with the abnormal ZZ allele never develop the disease.

- If you inherit one normal and one abnormal allele, as with phenotype MZ, for example, you are a carrier. Your risk for developing liver disease is much lower than the risk is for those with phenotype ZZ.

Here are two more terms that are useful to know:

- **Heterozygote.** This refers to a person who has two different alleles/genes. Examples would include MS, MZ, SZ. These people are generally carriers of the disorder but do not actually get the liver disease associated with deficiency. They have a 50/50 chance of passing the one abnormal gene/allele (S or Z) to their offspring, but since the offspring inherit their other gene from their spouse and this is likely to be the M allele, they too will be heterozygotes. Only when two abnormal genes come together do the offspring become homozygotes with a risk of disease. (See below.)

- **Homozygote.** This means that a person has two identical abnormal genes, such as SS or ZZ. The ZZ combination carries the greatest risk of disease.

Pediatric Liver Transplants

Nowadays, when a child's liver disease becomes severe, transplantation is a viable option with a very good chance of success. Biliary atresia creates by far the biggest need for pediatric transplants, but medical centers also see children with acute liver failure caused by A1AT deficiency, viral hepatitis, drug toxicity, neonatal iron-storage disease, tyrosinemia, and other illnesses. While encephalopathy in itself doesn't necessarily mandate a transplant, it is a frequent symptom in children who need to undergo transplants.

New hope also is seen for children with primary liver cancer. Increasingly they undergo transplantation in conjunction with chemotherapy and other treatments, with good outcomes. Compared to its frequency in the adult population, the appearance in children of HCC is relatively rare.

Interestingly, the age of the donor can be the critical factor in pediatric liver transplants. One study examined the database of the United Network for Organ Sharing (UNOS), and found that children who received liver transplants from other children had an 81 percent success rate (defined here as reaching the three-year mark), while children receiving transplants from adult donors did not fare quite so well. However, for obvious reasons livers from child donors are chronically in short supply. These days it is not uncommon for a child to receive part of a liver from a deceased adult, while an adult in need of a transplant receives the remainder of the liver. These "split livers" provide for the needs of both recipients.

LIVER DISEASE AND PREGNANCY

Sandra Clemens knew that she was gaining too much weight during her pregnancy, but the fact did not concern her greatly. It was her only chance to "eat for two," as her mother liked to say. Once the baby was born, resolved the 37-year-old cashier, she would get back to a healthier routine.

Working in a drugstore, Sandra had become fairly well informed about healthy practices for pregnant women. Information about nutrition, exercise, and the value of rest was all around her at work. And it wasn't as if she were doing anything dangerous to the baby, such as drinking wine (which she missed!) or smoking cigarettes. Still, she was indulging in pasta and desserts too often, and the pounds were piling on.

She had expected to gain extra weight. What she hadn't expected was to become seriously ill. About eight months into her pregnancy, Sandra started feeling nauseated. A few days later, when painful cramps began, she headed straight for the office of her OB-GYN.

It turned out that Sandra had developed acute fatty liver of pregnancy. She was smart to see her doctor right away, even before jaundice (a common symptom of this condition) had set in. Because the disease was caught early, more serious complications – such as encephalopathy and hypoglycemia – had not developed. Sometimes, when acute fatty liver occurs in pregnant women, they must undergo a liver transplant in order to survive.

Because Sandra had acted so quickly, an early delivery of her baby was sufficient treatment. (Fortunately, she wasn't suffering from any preexisting liver disease that required treatment.) Sandra experienced no lasting effects from the disease, and her liver began functioning normally again within a couple of weeks of her baby's delivery.

Diagnostic Dilemma

Whether a woman's liver disease is caused by her pregnancy or unrelated to it, it is just as difficult to diagnose as it is in other patients. Clues often are subtle or vague, and even the conventional liver tests can show unusual results because of the pregnancy. Some outward signs, such as spider angiomas (spider veins), are common in pregnant woman. Another sign, palmar erythema, sometimes called "liver palm," is characterized by red, blotchy palms; it, too, is common in pregnant women.

Once the dysfunction is recognized, appropriate diagnostic tests and treatment can save the lives of both mother and baby. The key is vigilance.

Liver Diseases Unique to Pregnant Women

A few liver diseases are seen only in pregnant women:

- **Hyperemesis gravidarum.** Severe nausea and vomiting are the more obvious symptoms of this unpleasant but usually harmless disease. Hyperemesis gravidarum usually disappears after the first trimester and does no lasting harm to mother or baby.

- **Acute fatty liver of pregnancy.** Usually seen in the third trimester, acute fatty liver of pregnancy causes abdominal pain, nausea, and vomiting at first; jaundice sets in a week or two later. Encephalopathy and hypoglycemia (low blood sugar) also develop, and the disease can be fatal. In some women, a prompt delivery restores liver function. For others, a transplant might be required.

- **Intrahepatic cholestasis of pregnancy.** The main symptom of this benign disorder is pruritus, or itching. While fetal distress has been reported with this disease – in which case prompt delivery might be necessary – the treatment usually consists only of ursodeoxycholic acid.

- **Preeclampsia and the HELLP syndrome.** These diseases often overlap in pregnant woman, so much so that most physicians regard the HELLP syndrome (hemolysis, elevated liver enzymes, and low platelets) as a consequence of preeclampsia and eclampsia. In preeclampsia, the woman develops hypertension and weight gain; as more serious eclampsia develops, she may experience seizures. Abdominal pain usually signals the development of the HELLP syndrome, a condition in which the mother's platelet count decreases dramatically. While some symptoms can be treated, the HELLP syndrome often requires early delivery.

Other Liver Diseases Affecting Pregnancy

Whether the mother has a preexisting liver disease or the liver dysfunction develops during her pregnancy, early detection and treatment are vital. A successful outcome also could depend on the severity of the disease, regardless of the pregnancy.

Liver disorders that can concern pregnant women include:

- **Portal hypertension and cirrhosis.** These are not common conditions among pregnant women, largely because they usually occur in women who are past their childbearing years or who are infertile because of the illness.

- **Autoimmune hepatitis and Wilson disease.** These diseases can be diagnosed for the first time during the pregnancy. Women previously diagnosed with autoimmune hepatitis can become pregnant and carry the child to full term, but the hepatitis must be closely monitored for possible complications. Women with Wilson disease also can have a successful pregnancy if the WD is identified and treated promptly. Medications have to be adjusted throughout the pregnancy, so close monitoring is essential.

> Whether the mother has a preexisting liver disease or the liver dysfunction develops during her pregnancy, early detection and treatment are vital.

- **Viral hepatitis.** There is a risk of transmission from mother to fetus, but it depends on the virus. Hepatitis A has no chronic form, so only an acute episode of hepatitis A would be an issue. This is rare, and if a pregnant woman does contract acute hepatitis A, it usually does not affect the fetus.

- **Chronic Hepatitis B.** This condition used to be a significant source of "vertical transmission" from mother to infant. Fortunately, an effective screening and vaccination program has virtually eliminated this type of transmission in the United States. The U.S. Centers for Disease Control now recommends that all pregnant women be screened for HBV and that all newborns receive the HBV vaccine.

- **Chronic hepatitis C.** If the mother is infected with hepatitis C, the rate of transmission to the fetus is quite low – less than 5 percent. That risk is higher if the mother also is co-infected with HIV. Also, interferon or pegylated interferon, a drug commonly used in treating hepatitis C, should not be taken during pregnancy. Ribavirin, another medication used to treat HCV, is well known to cause birth defects and absolutely should not be used during pregnancy or in women considering pregnancy. In fact, all women of childbearing age need to use effective contraception if they are to be considered for combination interferon/ribavirin treatment.

- **Hepatitis E.** Of all the forms of viral hepatitis, hepatitis E probably is the most dangerous to pregnant women, carrying a 25 percent rate of death. If they can possibly do so, pregnant women should avoid traveling to countries where hepatitis E is prevalent.

- **Alcoholic liver disease.** Even when pregnancy is not a factor, women are two to four times more likely to develop ALD than men drinking the same amount of alcohol. Women who drink during pregnancy increase the risk of miscarriage, stillbirth, premature delivery, retarded growth, and fetal alcohol syndrome, which can produce brain defects, cardiac defects, spinal defects, craniofacial abnormalities, and behavioral problems in their children. Pregnant women should eliminate the use of alcohol altogether.

TREATING PREGNANT WOMEN WITH LIVER DISEASE

When a doctor suspects liver disease in a pregnant patient, ultrasonography often is the first imaging choice because it is safe for the baby, as is magnetic resonance imaging (MRI). Depending on the illness, drug therapy may be called for, though many drugs that are commonly used in treating liver diseases have not been tested on pregnant women and have not been evaluated for ill effects on the unborn child. It is important that pregnant women consult a doctor with experience in treating pregnant liver patients, so that the relative benefits and risks of the diagnostic test and the medication in question can be explained.

There is no liver disease related to pregnancy that will prevent a woman from undertaking future pregnancies. However, knowledge of a previous pregnancy-related liver problem will alert both the patient and her obstetrician to be alert to possible future difficulties. Similarly, a liver transplant should not affect a woman's chances of becoming pregnant again in the future. For the optimum chance of success, it is generally recommended that she wait two years after the transplant to plan her next pregnancy. ◆

Chapter 13

Liver Testing Simplified

With more than two dozen different blood tests currently used to indicate specific liver functions and disorders – not to mention the popular imaging studies, such as sonograms, CT scans, and MRIs – for patients, the landscape of liver testing resembles a hopelessly confusing maze of high-tech jargon and initial-talk.

The liver is an unusually complex organ, responsible for filtering nearly every substance that comes into the body. As a result, it is vulnerable to a long list of potential hazards, from overloads of copper or iron to the "hepatitis alphabet."

Many liver tests, such as the liver function tests sometimes referred to as a hepatic function panel (HFP), cannot accurately diagnose diseases because the disorders themselves have so many shared features. What LFTs can do is to narrow the possibilities, advance the diagnostic procedures a step toward confirming the doctor's suspicions, and indicate which specialized tests the doctor and patient should undertake next. Imaging tests, too, can point the diagnostic team in the right direction. For some disorders, a more detailed scan, such as an MRI, can give a more definitive answer.

LIVER FUNCTION TESTS

As mentioned above, blood tests known as LFTs often do not pinpoint a specific disorder. What they do measure is how well the liver is doing in regard to particular functions and the levels of certain measurements associated with inflammation.

Dozens of different LFTs are performed in hospitals, but they all measure the levels of liver proteins, liver enzymes (called transaminases and cholestatic liver enzymes), and bilirubin.

TRANSAMINASES: AST AND ALT

LFTs that check the levels of AST (aspartate transaminase) and ALT (alanine transaminase) are looking for inflammation or injury to liver cells – in technical terms, hepatocellular liver injury. When the liver is damaged, AST and ALT often leak into the bloodstream, so they would be seen as *possible* indicators of liver damage. However, AST is also found in the heart, kidneys, and muscles, so elevated AST doesn't always mean a liver problem. But when it is coupled with elevated ALT, which *does* exist only in the liver, the higher AST level makes liver damage more probable.

The extent of the liver damage, though, cannot be determined by high transaminase levels alone. If a patient drinks alcohol a few hours before the blood test or works out in the gym the morning his or her blood is drawn, the transaminase levels may be mildly elevated. On the other hand, if alcohol abuse damaged the liver five years ago, the transaminase level may be normal, but still there could be some residual liver damage.

Moreover, men tend to have higher transaminase levels than women, and African American men usually show higher AST and ALT levels than Caucasian men. Almost everyone's transaminase levels are higher in the morning.

Obviously, high levels of AST and ALT should not be taken as certain signs of a serious liver disease. They are only the first clues along a path of diagnostic tests employed to pinpoint what is wrong. But while elevated transaminase levels might indicate strenuous exercise or recent alcohol use, they also could be caused by a fatty liver, alcoholic liver disease, viral hepatitis, autoimmune hepatitis, a genetic liver disease, a tumor, heart or lung failure, or some toxic injury to the liver.

CHOLESTATIC LIVER ENZYMES: GGTP AND AP

When the LFT indicates an elevated GGTP (gamma-glutamyl transpeptidase) and AP (alkaline phosphatase), suspicion falls on blocked, damaged, or inflamed bile ducts. When bile is not flowing adequately, a condition known as cholestatis develops. Any injury or illness involving bile ducts is known as a cholestatic liver injury or cholestatic liver disease.

When a doctor suspects intrahepatic cholestasis, it means that the blockage or damage is occurring in a bile duct *inside* the liver – a condition that can be found in patients with liver cancer or primary biliary cirrhosis – while extrahepatic cholestasis indicates an injury or blockage outside the liver. The bile backs up, the cholestatic enzymes GGTP and AP seep out into the bloodstream, and their levels may be very high. However, *both* GGTP and AP must be elevated in order to indicate a liver problem because while GGTP is mostly found in the liver, AP is routinely seen in the bones, kidneys, intestines, and placenta. For example, it is common to find an elevated AP during pregnancy or in an adolescent going through a growth spurt. In these circumstances, GGTP would be normal.

A few of the liver-related conditions that cause GGTP and AP to elevate include liver tumors, autoimmune hepatitis, nonalcoholic fatty liver disease, primary biliary cirrhosis, primary sclerosing cholangitis, and alcoholic liver disease, as well as gallstones – particularly those that may have moved out of the gallbladder.

BILIRUBIN

Usually associated with elevated GGTP and AP levels, bilirubin is the yellowish-green pigment that produces the condition known as jaundice. When the liver fails to excrete bilirubin, symptoms include a yellow cast to the skin and eyes; dark, tea-colored urine; and light-colored stools. Clearly, it is a dysfunction that is easy for a doctor and most people to spot.

High bilirubin levels, or jaundice, can be related to other conditions besides liver disease. When jaundice is present in a person with liver disease, it usually does signal cholestasis (blockage or injury to the bile ducts) or progression of the disease.

When elevated bilirubin is found alongside high levels of GGTP and AP, the patient is said to be cholestatic, and diseases linked to all three simultaneously elevated levels are cholestatic liver diseases. High bilirubin levels can be linked to alcoholic hepatitis, primary biliary cirrhosis, primary sclerosing cholangitis, gallstones in the bile duct, liver failure, tumors, viral hepatitis, a flare of autoimmune hepatitis, or a destruction of the red blood cells called hemolysis.

An elevated bilirubin also can indicate Gilbert syndrome, which is a common, benign, inherited condition of bilirubin uptake and metabolism by the liver. It is estimated that 6 to 10 percent of adults have the syndrome, though most are unaware of its presence. Usually, doctors discover it while screening for unrelated problems. When they include a bilirubin measurement, they find that the so-called unconjugated bilirubin is elevated. This is bilirubin before it has been metabolized by the liver. It is a completely harmless condition that has no clinical significance. It is not an indication for liver biopsy. There are no known complications and no treatment is needed.

LIVER PROTEINS

The liver produces many proteins – albumin, prothrombin, ceruloplasmin (containing copper). Sometimes inflammation in the liver stimulates the production of gamma globulin in other organs as well as in the liver. When the levels of these proteins are abnormal, it may signal disease in the liver.

A severely damaged liver cannot make albumin efficiently, so an abnormally low level of this protein, such as that found in patients with cirrhosis and chronic liver diseases, can point to liver damage. However, a malnourished person or someone otherwise in ill health might also lose the ability to produce albumin without experiencing a specific liver disease, so further tests are indicated to sort this out.

Prothrombin is a protein that the liver produces as one of the clotting factors that help stop bleeding. "Prothrombin time" (PT) is the time the body needs to begin clotting – normally between 9 and 11 seconds – and vitamin K must be present in order for clotting to happen. When vitamin K is deficient (which often happens with certain cholestatic liver diseases) or the liver has suffered extensive damage, the PT will be abnormally long, compromising the patient's ability to stop bleeding. Injections of vitamin K or oral supplementation sometimes help; when such an injection does help the PT return to normal, doctors know that the liver is working. If clotting does not improve after the vitamin K injection, the coagulopathy (inability to stop bleeding) might indicate liver disease.

The immunoglobulins are another group of liver-related proteins connected with the immune system. They are produced partly by the liver itself, but mostly by the immune system outside the liver. Many patients with chronic liver diseases display high levels of immunoglobulins. Specific immunoglobulins, such as IgA, IgG, and IgM, are possible indicators of specific liver diseases, mainly PBC and autoimmune hepatitis.

PLATELETS

In the clotting process, platelets are the actual blood cells that help form clots; they are stored in the spleen. In cirrhotic patients, the spleen becomes large because of portal hypertension (the blood backs up behind a scarred liver) and causes a condition known as splenomegaly, which traps the platelets. Low platelet levels are known as thrombocytopenia. When the spleen is enlarged and platelets are low, cirrhosis is a likely diagnosis – but, as with all laboratory measurements, further testing is necessary to confirm the diagnosis.

The table on page 141 is a list of blood tests used to confirm specific diagnoses that doctors may make after the first round of LFTs. It is a simple table – merely a list of liver diseases and blood tests commonly used to diagnose them – but it can be a handy reference in case your physician suspects any of these illnesses. Depending on the hospital, the laboratory, and the test itself, it can be anywhere from two days to two weeks before results of a given test are known. (The tests for Wilson disease and A1AT deficiency have been outlined in previous chapters.)

IMAGING STUDIES AND THE LIVER

After the medical team has collected the best chemical information from various blood tests, it is helpful for the doctors to be able to view the entire liver. They will look at its size, noting whether it has shrunk with scarring or grown larger, its location, and at any possible growths. They will also check for gallstones in the gallbladder.

The imaging studies performed on liver patients are sonograms (ultrasounds), computerized axial tomography scans (CT or CAT scans), and magnetic resonance imaging (MRIs). None of these procedures involves surgery, and all are performed while the patient is awake, often in a doctor's (radiologist's) office.

While most of us think of ultrasounds as the procedures done to allow a pregnant woman to see her fetus, they actually are the most frequently prescribed imaging studies used for liver patients. Unlike x-rays, sonograms use sound waves rather than radiation to show the image. Usually, the patient will have fasted for 12 hours so that the gallbladder will be full of bile, making it easy for the doctor to spot gallstones. Sonograms may also show tumors and estimate their size, though it is often impossible to tell with an imaging study whether the growth is benign or malignant. Sonograms are also often the first indication that a person has a fatty liver.

CT scans and MRIs are sometimes ordered to provide additional, more detailed images of the liver, especially when a tumor is suspected. Using radiation that sends an x-ray beam into the liver, a CT scan can identify abnormal growths (benign or malignant), while MRIs, using electromagnetic radiation, are helpful in identifying iron overload, hemangiomas (benign blood tumors), or sometimes a fatty liver.

BLOOD TESTS FOR SPECIFIC LIVER DISEASES

Disease	Test
Hepatitis A	◆ Hepatitis A antibody IgM and IgG (anti- HA Ab)
Hepatitis B	◆ Hepatitis B core antibody (HbcAb) ◆ Hepatitis B surface antigen (HbsAg) ◆ Hepatitis B surface antibody (HBsAb) ◆ Hepatitis B e antibody (HBeAb) ◆ Hepatitis B e antigen (HBeAg) ◆ Hepatitis B viral DNA (HBV-DNA)
Hepatitis C	◆ Hepatitis C virus antibody (anti-HCVAb) ◆ Hepatitis C virus ribonucleic acid (HCV-RNA) ◆ HCV-RNA Qualitative ◆ HCV RNA Quantitative (Viral Load) ◆ HCV RNA genotype (types 1-6)
Autoimmune Hepatitis	◆ Antinuclear antibody (ANA) ◆ Smooth muscle antibody (SMA) ◆ Anti-liver-kidney-microsomal antibody (LKMAb)
Primary Biliary Cirrhosis	◆ Antimitochondrial antibody (AMA) ◆ Elevated immunoglobulin M (IgM) (PBC)
Alcoholic Liver Disease	◆ Blood alcohol level ◆ Mean corpuscular volume (MCV) ◆ AST>ALT ◆ Vitamin B_{12} and Folate
Hemochromatosis	◆ Serum iron (Fe) ◆ Total iron binding capacity (TIBC) ◆ Percent transferrin saturation ◆ Serum ferritin ◆ Gene testing for hemochromatosis (HFE-DNA)
Liver Cancer (Hepatoma)	◆ Alpha-fetoprotein (AFP)

Even after a series of LFTs and imaging studies has been completed, doctors still may order a liver biopsy – the only test that can definitively diagnose certain serious but treatable liver diseases.

Liver specialists have been looking for an alternative to the traditional invasive liver biopsy, partly to satisfy the reluctance of some patients to undergo liver biopsy and partly to offer less invasive, less discomforting, and therefore safer means to detect scarring or cirrhosis. There has been some success in achieving this aim, but these tests are still in an early phase of development as noninvasive blood markers for liver fibrosis. These are blood tests that can identify the amount of fibrosis or scar tissue present in the liver. Unfortunately, thus far these tests have played only a limited role in clinical use. They are most useful in detecting the two extremes in the spectrum of liver fibrosis (i.e., very mild disease or very advanced disease). They are not very useful in identifying those patients with liver fibrosis that falls between the two extremes.

One novel additional noninvasive evaluation of liver fibrosis is transient elastography. Fibroscan is the commercial name for this technique, which is designed to measure liver stiffness. The machine measures the elasticity or stiffness of the liver and generates a report. The greater the degree of scarring, the less elastic the liver appears. Unfortunately, as with the blood markers mentioned above, this test does not appear to be accurate enough to replace the "gold standard" of the liver biopsy. Research continues, and hopefully the day will come when we will be able to replace the liver biopsy with a simple blood test or a simple, painless scan. ◆

Chapter 14

The Ultimate Liver Test: The Biopsy

When doctors order a liver biopsy, it is because they need a definitive answer about the type of problem affecting the liver and the extent of the damage it has caused. With that information, the patient's care team can plan a course of treatment, anticipate the body's probable response to that treatment, and form a prognosis. The liver biopsy is the only diagnostic test that can provide such accurate and complete information. For many liver diseases, all the tests that have been made to that point – blood work, imaging tests, and others – have given good supportive information but cannot accurately diagnose the extent of the problem.

Most liver diseases affect the entire organ, so in most cases, that one small piece provides all the information needed for a good diagnostic evaluation.

During a biopsy, a needle is used to remove a tiny sliver of the organ. The sample is about an inch long and looks like a piece of cord. It is sent to a laboratory, where its cells are examined. Most liver diseases affect the entire organ, so in most cases, that one small piece provides all the information needed for a good diagnostic evaluation. On rare occasions, the biopsy sample is not representative of the whole liver (this is known as a "sampling error") and the test may have to be performed again.

There are instances when a liver biopsy will not help doctors determine the best course of treatment. One is the case of a patient with acute hepatitis A; that patient would receive the same treatment regardless of the biopsy results, so the test is not recommended. Another is when a patient's liver disease is thought to have been caused by a medication; in that case, doctors would first cease giving that medication to see whether that resolves the problem without need for a biopsy.

Some liver patients are simply too ill to undergo a biopsy. Cirrhosis patients, for example, whose illness is complicated by ascites and coagulation problems, could risk excessive bleeding or infection. The biopsy would not be recommended in these circumstances.

BEFORE THE BIOPSY

As is the case before other diagnostic tests, the doctor should be alerted about all medications that the patient is taking, as well as about coexisting medical conditions that could affect the outcome of the

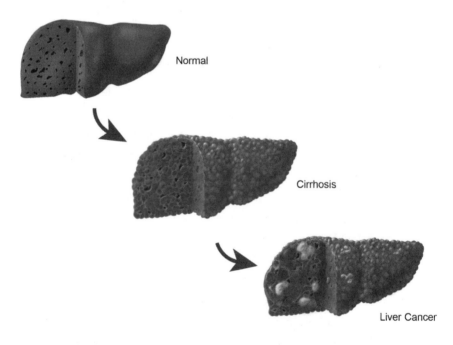

The outer surface of a normal liver is smooth. Cirrhosis results in scarring throughout the organ. When both cirrhosis and hepatocellular carcinoma are present, the liver also displays cancerous lesions.

biopsy. Because the liver is dense with blood vessels, there's always a small risk of bleeding associated with biopsies, so all medications and supplements that "thin" the blood (affecting its ability to clot) should be avoided for at least 10 days before the procedure. Also, most doctors will ask the patient to avoid eating or drinking for eight hours before the test.

Blood-thinners include medications such as Coumadin. Also to be avoided are nonsteroidal anti-inflammatory drugs (NSAIDs) such as ibuprofen (Advil, Motrin, Pamprin), aspirin, naproxen (Aleve), antiplatelet prescriptions (Plavix), and cyclooxygenase-2 (COX-2) inhibitors such as Celebrex. Small doses of acetaminophen (Tylenol) might be permissible, but the doctor must be consulted first.

Vitamin E and the many different vitamin formulations containing vitamin E should be discontinued a week before the biopsy because they could boost the effectiveness of aspirin and some blood-thinning drugs. Herbs such as garlic, ginseng, and ginkgo biloba could have the same effect and should be avoided as well.

One week to a month before the biopsy, the doctor will order blood work to evaluate the patient's risk of bleeding during the biopsy. Prothrombin time (PT), activated partial thromboplastin time (aPTT), and platelet count will be measured; if either shows a risk, doctors may order a transfusion of platelets or fresh frozen plasma (FFP) before the biopsy. Also, a sonogram will often be ordered as a precaution to check for any previously undiscovered liver mass or other abnormality.

Biopsies usually are outpatient procedures. Patients are required to remain in bed for two to six hours after the biopsy, so it is wise to take the precaution of using the lavatory right before the biopsy.

During the biopsy, the patient is asked to lie down, right arm up and resting behind the head, giving the doctor unobstructed access to the right upper abdomen. If the patient feels nervous, a mild sedative can be given, though it is best for the patient to remain awake during the test, since the doctor will ask for the breath to be held momentarily.

After the biopsy, the patient will lie on his back or right side for two to six hours while being monitored for the occurrence of any bleeding.

BIOPSY TECHNIQUES

For years, liver biopsies were performed using the "blind percutaneous stick" technique. In this straightforward test, the patient lies on his back, hand resting behind his head, while the doctor locates the liver by feel. After numbing the skin with a local anesthetic such as lidocaine, the doctor inserts a needle through the skin ("percutaneous") and draws out a small sample of liver tissue. The entire procedure takes only a few minutes, though the patient must lie still for two to six hours.

More common today is the ultrasound-guided biopsy. If the doctor wants to locate a liver mass or other precise area, the ultrasound – or, in some cases, a CT-guided biopsy – can guide the doctor to the spot in question. Guided biopsies also are helpful if the patient is overweight, making the liver difficult to locate, or if the gallbladder or intestines might be blocking the path to the liver. If the patient has advanced cirrhosis, the liver may have shrunk so much that it is difficult to locate without help from a scan of some sort.

If a patient is morbidly obese, has a problem with blood clotting, or has a very low platelet count, the doctor may call in a radiologist to perform a transvenous or transjugular liver biopsy. By this method a small tube is inserted into the jugular vein of the patient's neck and guided into the hepatic vein draining from the liver. The biopsy needle then follows the tube into the liver to retrieve the needed sample.

In some instances, the doctor will order a surgical biopsy known as a laparoscopic liver biopsy, usually performed in an operating room. Doctors insert a thin, lighted tube through an incision in the abdomen and direct the biopsy needle into that tube to obtain the biopsy sample.

COMPLICATIONS OF LIVER BIOPSIES

Although the possible complications from a liver biopsy sound ominous – bleeding, piercing nearby organs, and pain – the good news is that less than 1 percent of patients who undergo a liver biopsy report any complications at all. With ultrasound-guided biopsies, the rate is negligible.

A small amount of bleeding after a liver biopsy is common and is not a cause for worry. If excessive bleeding occurs, it is likely to happen within a few hours of the biopsy and usually can be resolved with blood transfusions and close monitoring.

Because the human body is packed quite densely, it is possible that even an experienced doctor can puncture a nearby organ – usually a kidney, lung, or colon – by mistake. The tiny hole made by the biopsy needle usually heals by itself, though the patient will be kept in the hospital until the healing is accomplished. Occasionally, the gallbladder will be punctured, causing a small leak of bile into the abdomen. Such a leak can cause peritonitis, an inflammation of the abdominal fluid, and calls for intravenous antibiotic treatment and monitoring.

About one-third of patients describe their post-biopsy pain as similar to being hit in their side or stomach. When that occurs, the doctor will recommend a small dose of acetaminophen, but caution against taking NSAIDs or aspirin for a week. If the post-biopsy pain is still present after 24 hours, the patient should return to the hospital immediately.

AFTER A BIOPSY

Biopsies are not major surgeries, and patients need not plan a long recuperation. They're advised to rest for a day and avoid driving, dancing, and sports for 24 hours. After a day, they can remove the small dressing, shower, and carry on their normal routines. Those with physically strenuous jobs should take it easy for an extra day or two before resuming any rigorous activity. Unless a symptom appears, such as shortness of breath, fever, chills, abdominal distention, or severe pain, there should be no aftereffects from a liver biopsy at all. In general, it is a quick and relatively painless test. ◆

Chapter 15

Liver Transplants

Scott knew for a long time that a liver transplant would be the outcome of his long battle with liver disease. The 45-year-old high school math teacher had been diagnosed with primary sclerosing cholangitis (PSC), a disease of the liver and bile ducts, more than five years earlier. His treatments had included balloon dilation of the ducts, but he also was suffering complications from the lack of bile flow through the ducts – pruritus (itching), serious deficiencies of fat-soluble vitamins, and, most recently, the onset of severe fatigue. It was time to move on a liver transplant.

Fortunately, Scott's physician had had the foresight to talk with his patient about a living-donor liver transplant. Scott was an only child, but a number of his fellow teachers and even the principal at his school volunteered to have their blood and livers tested. One of Scott's colleagues, a 34-year-old track coach named Ned, was selected as the best donor.

As "transplant day" approached, both Scott and Ned became minor celebrities in their town. Friends and strangers alike wished them well, and their students made videos to cheer them through their recuperation.

As expected, the surgery was successful – though Ned had a scare when doctors discovered a number of small bile leaks from the remaining portion of his liver. They assured him it was a common post-surgical complication of living donations, but they monitored him closely to be sure it resolved on schedule. Two months later, Ned was back in the classroom, and Scott followed him back to school the following month.

A HISTORY OF SUCCESS

Although we still view organ transplants as somewhat exotic procedures, the fact is that liver transplants have been around for about 40 years. Since the first successful transplant was performed in 1968, such surgeries have become almost routine and been accompanied by increasingly predictable success, with some transplant patients now having survived two decades or more after their surgeries. In the vast majority of cases, the patients lead normal lives, not at all deterred from vigorous work and play.

About 5,000 liver transplants now are performed in the United States each year, at more than 125 transplant centers. While doctors don't place the patient's name on the transplant list too far in advance, they also don't want to wait until the disease is so advanced that the patient might not survive the wait for the new liver.

A general guideline indicates that the time has come for referral when doctors estimate that the patient cannot live more than two years without a new liver. Indications of liver failure (such as worsening jaundice) or of advanced cirrhosis (such as ascites or encephalophathy) will justify a referral, and patients whose chronic liver disease has progressed to liver cancer also should be evaluated for a transplant. Physicians also order evaluations when the patient's symptoms, such as pruritus or fatigue, are dramatically affecting the patient's quality of life, even if the disease itself may not have progressed to the transplant stage.

There are some patients, unfortunately, who will not qualify for a transplant because they exhibit certain conditions, known as *absolute* contraindications, which probably would prevent the transplant's success. Among the absolute contraindications are serious heart or lung disease, active uncontrolled infection, active alcohol or drug abuse, AIDS (but not HIV), metastatic liver cancer (i.e., liver cancer that has spread to other parts of the body), and cancer elsewhere that did not originate in the liver.

Other patients might be seen as borderline candidates for success if they display *relative* contraindications. They are not necessarily denied referrals for a new liver, but they are evaluated very carefully and may or may not be granted a transplant if they exhibit morbid obesity, failed kidneys, advanced age (older than 70 years, with disease of other organs), previous cancer in any organ, malnutrition, HIV, extensive portal vein thrombosis (a blood clot in the portal vein), or a failure thus far to adhere to physicians' medication or wellness regimens.

BEFORE THE TRANSPLANT

The doctor's approval is only the first step toward obtaining a new liver. The patient then meets the transplant team – liver specialists (hepatologists), a transplant surgeon, anesthesiologist, a social worker, a psychiatrist, and possibly other doctors, such as heart or lung specialists, depending on the patient's condition – and is evaluated by them as well. Additional MRIs and diagnostic tests such as a colonoscopy, blood tests, and upper endoscopy (to check for esophageal varices) are ordered, and if the medical team concludes that the patient is a suitable candidate for a transplant, he or she is added to a waiting list.

As of 2002, the system for distributing new livers was revised. The old system had been widely criticized because of the public's perception of an appearance of inequalities based on fame and or financial status. The new system, the Model for End-Stage Liver Disease (MELD), is a mathematical "score" that does not recognize celebrity or favoritism. Instead, the MELD score calculates the severity of the patient's liver disease on the basis of the mathematical probability (derived from the results of three blood tests) of the patient's dying within three months without a transplant. Those with liver cancer receive a different MELD score, measuring the status of the cancer. Simply put, the sickest patient gets the new liver.

During the waiting period, patients should stay as active as possible because their strength and stamina will be a tremendous help to them in their recovery.

Patients who are not hospitalized while waiting for a liver are asked to carry a beeper or a cellular phone so the transplant team can notify them immediately when a liver is found. The transplant center performing the surgery must accept the liver within one hour, and if its staff cannot contact the patient, they will call (or beep) the next patient on the list. If the transplant recipient is feeling well when the call comes, with no fever or signs of a developing illness, then he or she should proceed to the transplant center immediately. Considerations such as babysitters, pet care, transportation to the hospital, and a packed suitcase should be arranged in advance so that the patient can leave at a moment's notice.

In the case of complete transplants – that is, when the donor's entire liver is transplanted into the recipient – the donor will be a newly deceased, brain-dead person with a healthy heart and circulatory system. A family member of the donor will have signed a consent form for the donation. However, even if the donor had, in life, indicated a wish to donate his or her liver, several factors can prevent the donation: If the prospective donor has been diagnosed with cancer, AIDS, or active hepatitis B, or tests positive for HIV, then that person's liver cannot be used. In addition, the donor's liver function tests should typically be in the normal range, and the liver shouldn't contain more than 30 percent fat, as fatty livers typically are rejected by the body shortly after the transplant. The donor should be relatively young (under 60, if possible) and the body size and blood type should be similar to the recipient's. Livers from donors up to age 70 have been successfully transplanted, as have those from donors who have been diagnosed with hepatitis C, if the recipient also is a hepatitis C patient.

It is a complex undertaking to manage the waiting list, recover and transport organs very quickly, and protect the organs until they can be transplanted. The entity responsible for accomplishing those tasks is the Organ Procurement Organization (OPO), the primary link between an organ donor and the recipient.

Each OPO is assigned a geographic area. When an organ is about to become available, the hospital notifies the OPO, which then scans the database and matches the donated organ with a recipient. Some patients are listed at more than one transplant center – a "multiple listing"– so that they can be considered for organs that become available in adjacent areas; in these instances, the OPOs involved manage coordination between their areas.

In addition to its fast and efficient work when a transplant is imminent, the OPO also works to educate the public and health-care providers about the need for donating organs and tissue.

LIVING-DONOR LIVER TRANSPLANTS

Thanks to medical advances in recent years, it is now possible to obtain a liver transplant from a living donor – in fact, about 22 percent of the 5,000 liver transplants in the United States each year involve living donors.

Here's how living-donor transplants work: The patient's diseased liver is removed, while a piece of the donor's liver also is cut from the healthy liver in a separate surgery. Immediately, the healthy tissue is implanted in the patient.

This innovative technique is possible because the liver is able to regenerate, or regrow, when part of it has been cut away. Usually, the regeneration happens very quickly – in six to eight weeks at most. Within that time, both the donor and the recipient will have normal-sized, healthy livers again.

The greatest advantage of a living-donor liver transplant is that doctors can arrange the transplant when it is medically necessary, rather than having to wait for a liver from a deceased donor. Too often, liver patients languish on the waiting list for so long that, by the time a liver becomes available, they are too sick to undergo the transplant or even die before they can get a new liver. If their condition worsens while they wait, their recovery will be more difficult, with greater likelihood of complications.

In living-donor transplants, the incisions for both donor and recipient are large, but they should heal quickly. Up to 60 percent of the donor's healthy liver is removed – usually part of the right lobe, but in some cases the smaller left lobe plus a small part of the right lobe. Donors will have been informed that they will experience quite a bit of postoperative pain. Pain medications will be prescribed after surgery, but often in appropriately smaller doses that can be handled by their regenerating liver.

ADDITIONAL TRANSPLANT PROCEDURES

Depending on their conditions, patients may have more choices than a liver transplanted from a deceased donor or a liver transplanted from a living donor. One of the most promising new developments, in fact, takes the transplant concept to a new level: split-liver transplantation.

With a split-liver transplant, one whole, healthy liver from a deceased donor is divided into two portions, with the two "halves" given to different patients. In some instances, a larger portion is transplanted into an adult, while a child or smaller adult can receive the smaller part. The clear advantage of split-liver transplantation is the maximal use of each available liver, so that patients don't have to wait so long for their transplants and so that for children in particular, the wait for a deceased, child-sized liver can be avoided. Thus far, survival rates in these surgeries are comparable to rates for patients with conventional transplants.

In auxiliary transplants, surgeons transplant a small piece of donor liver into a patient who has experienced liver failure. The patient's diseased liver is kept intact. Reports on the success of auxiliary transplants are sketchy, and the procedure needs further study.

Even less is known about hepatocyte transplantation, a procedure in which a donor's liver cells (hepatocytes) are injected into a patient suffering from a genetic liver defect or sudden liver failure. Much of the research to date has been performed on animals, but the results are encouraging.

Gene therapy, too, might prove a useful tool in the future treatment of liver disease. Scientists have developed the ability to take samples of liver cells, manipulate the genes, and insert the modified cells back into the genetically defective liver. However, the long-term effectiveness of this technique has not yet been established. Gene therapy might also be valuable in preventing rejections of transplanted livers.

For those patients with sudden liver failure, an invention known as a liver-assist device has been explored for use as a temporary treatment. Essentially a liver-dialysis machine, the liver-assist can remove liver toxins in the short term, "buying" time for those who are awaiting a liver transplant within a few days. The success of liver-assist devices remains very limited at the time of this writing.

WHAT TO EXPECT AFTER THE TRANSPLANT

Once the surgery is completed, one of the patient's major concerns is whether the new liver will be accepted and functional. If the patient's immune system attacks the new liver (a process known as rejection), it may become temporarily compromised. Such episodes of acute rejection are usually overcome with additional immunosuppressants, strong medications that assist the body in accepting a new liver. In recent years the rate of rejection has declined, thanks to those same immunosuppressants. An exact figure would be difficult to pinpoint, as there persists a wide variation in the incidence of acute rejection reported by different studies. For essentially all transplant patients, immunosuppressant therapy is a lifelong endeavor.

In combating rejection, doctors have a number of immunosuppressant medications from which to choose, although none is without side effects. Cyclosporine is sometimes used, but the drug can carry serious side effects. It changes the metabolism of sugar and fat in the body, putting the patient at higher risk of hypertension and heart disease, and it can affect the central nervous system.

Tacrolimus is another immunosuppressive drug approved by the FDA, but it, too, is associated with possible serious side effects, including kidney and neurological damage, loss of alertness, hypertension, high cholesterol, and possibly development of diabetes.

A common post-transplant medication is prednisone, a corticosteroid that has both anti-inflammatory and immunosuppressive properties. While prednisone was once given to transplant patients for life, it has been shown that patients now can withdraw from the drug after about three months without affecting survival or acceptance of the new liver.

Some transplant patients experiencing rejection of the new liver or suffering severe side effects from cyclosporine or tacrolimus are given mycophenolate mofetil, an effective immunosuppressant. While it can bring about lower levels of both white and red blood cells, this drug has proved valuable in transplant-rejection management. Another drug sometimes used is sirolimus, which is reported to have less kidney toxicity but carries its own set of potential side effects. These problems appear to be diminished if sirolimus use is begun later after transplantation.

Overall, liver transplantation is a very successful treatment for end-stage liver disease that can no longer be managed medically, with about 90 percent of patients exhibiting no serious problems within the first year of receiving their new livers. After 10 years, approximately 55 percent of transplant patients are still alive and have a good quality of life.

After transplantation, recurrence of liver disease is a strong possibility for patients whose transplants were necessitated by chronic hepatitis C. This is a problem that is receiving a great deal of research attention in transplant centers around the world. Recurrence of a few other diseases – PSC and PBC – has been reported but is relatively infrequent.

For most patients, life and a return to normal health can be expected after a transplant. Women of childbearing age can become pregnant a year after receiving their new livers and most patients can return to their previous occupations. Quality of life can be high – especially for patients who commit to managing their health with diet and exercise, and careful adherence to their prescribed medications. Of course, regular follow-up by the transplant team will also help to ensure such a life-preserving and -enhancing outcome. ◆

Chapter 16

Nontraditional Therapies, Alternative Medicine, and Spirituality

It is no secret that alternative medicine is an enormously popular choice in health care, not only with Americans but with people all over the world. Herbal treatments, vitamin therapies, and dietary supplements have launched careers and boosted book sales for renowned authors such as Dr. Andrew Weil, and some of the most successful magazines on the newsstands, including *Prevention, Yoga Journal, Natural Health,* and *Body + Soul,* publish health-related articles with a holistic or natural approach. Even Cleveland Clinic now has a Department of Integrative Medicine for the study and use of alternative health-care therapies.

Today the buzz word is "integrative" medicine, rather than "alternative." (Even the famous Dr. Weil, an M.D., refers to the practice of nonconventional medicine in this way.) The message is that herbs, vitamins, and supplements can be *integrated* into one's health-care regimen, but they should not be an alternative to accepted medical practices.

SPECIAL NUTRITION NOTES

We will detail the basics of a liver-healthy diet in Chapter 17, but any discussion of integrative medicine should include some nutritional guidelines as well. In general, a liver-healthy diet would include between 60 percent and 70 percent complex carbohydrates – think whole-grain bread and whole-wheat pasta – and no more than 30 percent protein, as lean as possible. Only a small percentage of the diet (as little as 10 percent) should come from fats, and drinking eight glasses of water a day is a good habit for almost everyone.

Here are some other nutrition pointers for liver patients:

- Eliminate alcohol from your diet altogether.

- Avoid processed foods.

- Don't give up coffee! That may sound counterintuitive, in light of all the negatives we've heard about caffeine over the years. But new evidence shows that for patients at risk of developing chronic liver disease, as little as two cups of coffee a day can lower risk – and the inverse relationship between coffee drinking and HCC (hepatocellular carcinoma, or liver cancer) is especially strong.

- Build as many fresh fruits and vegetables into your daily diet as possible.

Talk to your doctor about taking the best combination of vitamins and antioxidants for you. Most multivitamins contain iron, which liver patients should avoid, and might not contain enough of other substances that would be beneficial.

HERBS THAT LOVE YOUR LIVER

The first thing to know about herbal treatments for the liver is this: What we *don't* know about herbal medicine could fill an ocean. Herbal medicine is not regulated by the Food and Drug Administration, and most herbal concoctions have not undergone the rigorous clinical studies to which prescription medicines are subjected. In fact, many available herbs can be harmful, especially when taken with other medications.

For instance, licorice root is widely used in Japan to treat liver problems; it is believed to lower transaminase levels. Yet, some research indicates it could cause fluid retention, thereby contributing to high blood pressure in some patients.

That said, several herbs are increasingly accepted by the medical community as beneficial to the liver:

Milk thistle is one of the best-known herbal treatments for the liver. In its seeds are found three substances collectively called silymarin, an antioxidant believed to fight toxins and pollutants. Sold in Germany as a supplemental treatment for chronic liver disease, milk thistle was found in recent European studies to help in treating alcoholic cirrhosis and aid recovery from hepatitis. It also is a tool in fighting the severe poisoning that results from consumption of the "death cap" mushroom (Amanita phalloides). Readers should note, however, that while milk thistle might help in lowering elevated liver enzyme levels, it cannot cure the hepatitis B or C viruses.

Milk thistle is not easily water-soluble, so the most effective method of ingesting this herb is in capsule form. There is no standardized dosage, but various experts recommend dosages from 70 to 2,000 mg, two to three times per day. Its side effects are rare and usually mild, and include joint pain, headache, stomach upset, hives, itching, and nausea.

Licorice is sometimes mentioned as beneficial to liver patients, but its effectiveness is not proven – and its side effects can be serious. In addition to water retention, licorice can generate low potassium levels and high blood pressure, and patients with chronic hepatitis, cholestatic liver disease, and cirrhosis are strongly advised against using it. Moreover, licorice can contain iron, making it dangerous for patients with hemochromatosis, and it could interact badly with prednisone, a steroid drug used to treat autoimmune hepatitis and as an immunosuppressant after a liver transplant. Licorice also can decrease testosterone levels and counteract the diuretic used in treating ascites.

Artichokes are another liver-friendly plant, with benefits that are similar to but not as strong as those offered by milk thistle. They are a great source of fiber, vitamin C, potassium, and folic acid. The helpful ingredient in artichoke leaves is called cynarin. If you read the

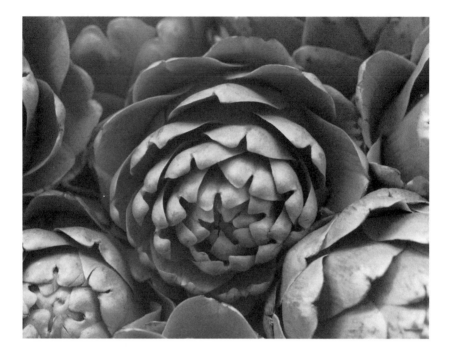

labels of many liver-detox supplements in health-food stores, you will find that artichoke-leaf extract is listed as an ingredient, often in combination with milk-thistle seed, selenium, and "bitter herbs" believed to be liver-friendly such as dandelion root (or greens), chard, and arugula.

Siberian ginseng (also known as eleuthero) is said to stimulate the immune system and boost energy as a general tonic. Its benefit for the liver, according to a Korean study, derives chiefly from the polysaccharides, substances in the stem that reduce enzyme levels. Side effects are rare, but include drowsiness, headache, irritability, anxiety, and depression. Pregnant or nursing women should avoid eleuthero, as should anyone with hypertension.

Green tea contains large concentrations of catechin, an antioxidant substance that helps to protect cell membranes, thereby making it similar to milk thistle, in theory, as a liver-friendly plant. This claim has not been proven in laboratory studies, though the antioxidant properties of green tea are a fact. (Black tea contains much less catechin than its green counterpart.)

Turmeric, a key ingredient in Indian curry powder, has been used for centuries by Ayurvedic medicine practitioners in fighting liver disease. Its yellow pigment, curcumin, is believed to be effective in fighting liver toxins, but that claim has not been proven in clinical studies.

SUBSTANCES TO AVOID

While little has been documented regarding herbal treatments that benefit the liver, we know a great deal more about substances that might harm the liver. This list is not complete, but the following have been linked to liver damage and disease, and should be avoided by liver patients:

- Black cohosh
- Buckthorn
- Chaparral, also known as greasewood and creosote bush
- Comfrey, germander
- Kava kava
- Kombucha
- Lobelia
- Ma huang, or ephedra
- Maté
- Mistletoe
- Nutmeg
- Pennyroyal
- Pokeweed
- Ragwort
- Sarsaparilla
- Sassafras
- Saw palmetto
- Skullcap
- Soy phytoestrogen
- Sweet clover
- Tansy
- Valerian
- Woodruff

SPIRITUALITY

Historically, spirituality has been intimately connected with medicine in many different cultures. This fusion has been promoted by such spiritual leaders as medicine men, witch doctors, ministers, shamans, rabbis, mullahs, priests, and "holy men."

Until very recently, religion and spirituality have been largely banished from "modern" medicine. This seems ironic, since recent Gallup polls have repeatedly found that around 95 percent of the U.S. population claims a belief in God and about 85 percent considers religion important to daily life.

It must be stated that spirituality and religion or religiosity are not the same thing. This can be a sticking point for many people and must to be clarified. For our purposes, spirituality can be defined broadly as a belief in something greater than oneself and the recognition that there is meaning to existence that transcends one's immediate circumstances.

Characteristics that are commonly attributed to spirituality include a diminished focus on the self, empathy, compassion, selflessness, and gratitude. Religiousness or religiosity usually refers to the practices and/or beliefs of a specific religion or religious group. When one conducts research into spirituality, significant numbers of people must be included to produce meaningful results. Therefore, most large studies are focused on cohorts of people who regularly attend religious services. These people are assumed to have spirituality. This does not mean that nonreligious attendees do not have spirituality; it just means that researchers needed to find large, relatively homogenous groups to study.

Spirituality is a concept that can be quite difficult to measure on an individual basis as there is no simple blood test that one can order. In fact, before the year 2000 nearly 1,200 studies around the world had examined the relationship between spirituality and health. The overwhelming majority of these studies showed a positive benefit between spirituality and health. Some of these earlier studies and their findings were criticized for having a poor study design and for other reasons. This prompted researchers to prospectively evaluate the role of spirituality on health in an expanded fashion that was more academically rigorous.

Two large recent studies of more than 4,000 participants revealed essentially the same findings as were reported earlier. People who regularly attended religious services had better health-related outcomes than those who did not show regular attendance. This means that people who regularly attended religious services had fewer

THE LATEST ON ACETAMINOPHEN

Because acetaminophen is an over-the-counter pain reliever (most popularly sold as Tylenol), most Americans are sometimes unaware of its potential danger to the liver.

Each year, acetaminophen overdoses send thousands of people to hospital emergency rooms, and hundreds of them die. It is the top cause of death in this country's poison-control centers, and some studies show it is the most frequent cause of acute liver failure.

An accidental overdose is an easy mistake to make, since about 45 million people, or one-fifth of American adults, take acetaminophen every week. About 7 million of them are under 18 years of age.

If you need to use a painkiller for headaches, joint aches or other ailments, be sure to talk with your doctor before using acetaminophen – and, if you choose to take it, read the label carefully and never exceed the recommended dosage. In fact, Tylenol (acetaminophen) is one of the safest pain medications often used in patients with chronic liver disease. The caveat is that no alcohol should be consumed and that appropriate dosing guidelines must be followed. Each patient is different and should discuss this with a specialist in hepatology.

mental-health issues, fewer substance-abuse problems, and fewer chronic diseases, and made less use of health-care services. They also had improved overall survival rates. One striking example of this finding was that African Americans who regularly attended religious services lived an average of 14 years longer than those who did not.

We are now seeing a resurgence of spirituality in medicine. Undoubtedly this is in direct response to the current high-tech, impersonal, and hurried medical environment that is leaving patients feeling disillusioned. There is no shortage of current popular literature supporting spirituality and health. More important, sound scientific experiments are under way that will undoubtedly continue to validate the crucial role of spirituality in health.

Members of the general public or medical profession who continue to ignore the spiritual dimensions of health are ignoring a possible dimension of healing and maintenance of well-being. The concept of spirituality has unexplored potential for empowering individuals to achieve improved physical and social well-being. ◆

Chapter 17

The Liver-Healthy Lifestyle

It is not difficult to design a diet, exercise, and lifestyle plan that will benefit the liver. Make healthy choices all day long, and with just a bit of fine-tuning, your healthy lifestyle also will benefit your liver as well as your other organs and psychological well-being.

LIFESTYLE NO-BRAINERS

No longer does anyone argue that smoking can be part of a healthy life. The harm it inflicts on our lungs and heart is well documented. What isn't as well known is the damage that smoking can do to the liver.

In essence, smoking robs the liver of its ability to do its job. We depend on the liver to process any drugs, alcohol, environmental toxins, and other harmful substances that we take into our bodies. Research shows that smoking damages the liver's capacity to detoxify those dangerous substances and remove them from our bodies, especially if the smoker already has been diagnosed with chronic hepatitis C. Some data also shows that smoking can accelerate existing liver disease, particularly if that disease was caused by alcohol.

It cannot be overemphasized that alcohol is toxic to the liver. Even in a healthy person, drinking to excess can cause liver disease. Anyone with alcohol-related liver disease should avoid drinking altogether, as should patients with hepatitis B or C. The most prudent course for anyone diagnosed with any liver disease is to stop consuming alcohol, though in some cases an occasional drink on a special occasion might be permissible and will not cause a sudden relapse.

A LIVER-HEALTHY DIET

Everyone has read that a low-fat, low-carbohydrate, high-fiber diet is good for the heart. That same balance is good for the liver: A heart-healthy diet is a liver-healthy diet.

The liver is critical to our nutritional well-being. It is the organ that refines and purifies everything we eat, breathe, and even absorb through our skin; the American Liver Foundation refers to it as our body's "internal chemical power plant." It converts our food into stored energy, removes alcohol and toxic substances from the blood, processes drugs absorbed from the digestive system so the body can use them effectively, and manufactures important chemicals the body needs, including bile.

About 90 percent of the blood leaving the digestive system carries nutrients to the liver to be converted for other body functions. It stores carbohydrates (or sugars) and releases them as energy when the body needs them. It also releases amino acids, the building blocks for proteins, to the muscles, and when some of the proteins are converted into ammonia, the liver breaks it down and converts it to urea so that it can be excreted by the kidneys.

The liver also produces bile – think of it as a kind of detergent – which breaks apart fat into tiny droplets; it also is vital for the body's absorption of vitamins A, D, E, and K. Also, it is not always appreciated that through its production of bile the liver is the main route for excretion of cholesterol from the body as well as a main site for its manufacture. While poor nutrition won't cause liver disease, it definitely does not help the liver to stay healthy.

Fortunately, the U.S. Department of Agriculture (USDA) has eliminated the need for guesswork in planning good nutrition. The agency defines a "healthy diet" as one that:

- Emphasizes fruits, vegetables, whole grains, and fat-free or low-fat milk and milk products
- Includes lean meats, poultry, fish, beans, eggs, and nuts
- Is low in saturated fats, trans fats, cholesterol, sodium, and added sugars

Within that very broad framework, it is fairly easy to create an eating plan with plenty of room for customization. Take yogurt – please. For more than a century, we've known that the probiotics (live bacteria used in the fermentation of dairy products to make yogurt) are a natural boost for the immune system. Low in fat and packed with calcium and protein, yogurt is an almost perfect food. Anyone who doesn't care for the taste can add some fresh fruit or sugar-free jam for a sweeter snack.

In 2005, the USDA revised its dietary guidelines for all adults, making it easier than ever to plan a healthy, tasty food program. They include the following suggestions:

- Consume 2 cups of fruit and 2 1/2 cups of vegetables per day.
- Consume 3 or more ounces of whole-grain products per day.
- Consume 3 cups per day of fat-free or low-fat milk or milk products per day.
- Consume less than 10 percent of calories from saturated fatty acids, and keep trans fat consumption as low as possible.
- Try to get your fats from fish, nuts, and vegetable oils.
- Choose lean, low-fat, or fat-free meats, poultry, dry beans, milk, and milk products.
- Choose fiber-rich fruits, vegetables, and whole grains.
- Prepare foods and beverages with minimal added sugars or sweeteners and starches.
- Consume fewer than 2,300 milligrams of sodium (about 1 teaspoon of salt) per day.
- Consume alcohol in moderation, if at all (up to one drink per day for women, two for men).

The USDA's dietary guidelines website, www.mypyramid.gov, offers much more detail regarding food choices and their implications. You can see, for instance, the various categories of vegetables – dark green, orange, dry beans and peas, starchy, and others – with long lists of specific vegetables for each category and recommendations for amounts men and women should consume each week. Furthermore, confusing terms such as whole grains, refined grains, and oils are discussed at length.

Another useful resource for learning and following a liver-healthy diet is the website of the American Heart Association (www.american heart.org). Remember, a heart-healthy diet is a liver-healthy diet. The AHA recommends these six easy-to-follow steps in making food choices:

- **Choose and prepare foods with little or no salt.** The sodium in table salt can make you retain fluids, and fluid retention is unhealthy for both liver and heart patients. As you plan your meals, keep the number 2,300 in your mind, and try to take in no more than 2,300 milligrams of sodium each day. These days, it's not difficult to cut salt from your diet. Read food labels carefully and look for tasty salt-free or low-sodium substitutes. Even beef, chicken, and vegetable broth is available salt-free.

- **Choose lean meats and poultry without skin, and prepare them without added saturated and trans fat.** If you cook chicken or other meat to mix into a salad or pasta, spray your frying pan with a spray flavored with olive oil instead of frying the meat in oil or butter. The strong, delicious flavor will surprise you.

- **Buy low-fat dairy products.** Milk, butter, and many cheeses are now produced with little fat. For a high-protein snack, try low-fat string cheese.

- **Try to eliminate drinks with added sugars.**

- **Cut back on foods high in dietary cholesterol.** Set a goal of less than 300 milligrams of cholesterol each day.

- **Watch your portion sizes, especially when eating out.**

HOW MUCH IS TOO MUCH?

Doctors, nurses, nutritionists, and other health professionals all agree: Americans eat too much. If there's one thing we need to learn in order to maintain a healthy weight, it is portion control – but exactly what is a reasonable portion?

DIET AND ENCEPHALOPATHY

When a diseased liver cannot clear away toxins from the bloodstream, a condition known as encephalopathy develops. With encephalopathy, the patient's symptoms range from mood swings to severe confusion, drowsiness, and coma.

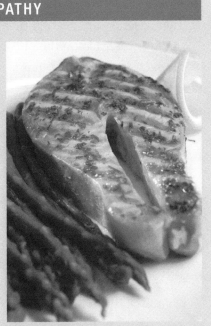

Certain foods can aggravate or help symptoms of encephalopathy. The two most important rules for a patient to follow are:

- **Avoid red meat as much as possible.**

- **Eat 80 grams of protein a day** to maintain good muscle mass. Non-meat protein sources include tofu, beans, and fish. You can also find protein powders at health-food stores that easily blend into drinks. (Most of these protein substitutes are soy-based or wheat-based.)

In addition, some encephalopathy patients display low levels of zinc; for those individuals, a doctor might recommend zinc supplements.

Sometimes, the answer is found on the food label – the U.S. FDA's "Nutrition Facts." That chart, found on most packaged foods, tells us how much fat, protein, calories, fiber, and other nutrients are found in a certain amount of the food inside the package. It refers to the amount being measured for nutrients as one "serving."

The American Heart Association advises all consumers to read nutrition labels as they shop for groceries, paying special attention to the following:

- **Serving size.** All food labels list the size of one serving and the nutrients contained in that amount. If you eat double the serving size listed on the nutrition label, you are eating twice as much fat, calories, sodium, and other nutrients as you see listed for one serving.

- **Calories.** If you are trying to lose weight, you must expend more calories each day than you take in, so this number obviously is important.

- **Total fat.** Even if you're not trying to lose weight, it is important not to consume a fatty diet if you want to keep your heart and liver functioning optimally. Nutrition labels give the number of grams of fat per serving, so that we can track our daily fat intake and the number of calories from fat in each serving. Overweight persons should obtain no more than 30 percent of their total calories from fat.

- **Saturated fat.** It is important to eat as little saturated fat as possible, since saturated fat raises the level of blood cholesterol and increases a person's risk of heart disease and stroke.

- **Cholesterol.** Aim for less than 300 mg of cholesterol each day, to keep your blood "lean" and help prevent heart disease and strokes.

- **Sodium.** This may be the sneakiest measure on a nutrition label, because many packaged foods – even so-called diet foods – contain high amounts of sodium, or salt. Keep your daily total to less than 2,300 mg of sodium, the equivalent of about one teaspoon of salt.

- **Total carbohydrate.** Try to get as many carbohydrates as possible from whole-grain breads and cereals, vegetables, and fruits. "Dense carbs," such as those found in bagels, white breads, and baked goods, can contribute to insulin resistance and consequently fatty liver disease. The latter group also depletes your energy and makes you sluggish, so the more you can avoid them, the better you'll feel during the day.

- **Protein.** Animal protein is almost always fatty. We need protein to build muscle, but try to keep it lean, from chicken, turkey, lean seafoods, and beans.

- **Daily Value.** The values cited on nutrition labels are intended to guide individuals who eat about 2,000 calories each day. If you eat fewer calories, or more, your daily value could be higher or lower. When you choose foods each day, keep in mind the number of calories you should be eating in order to reach or maintain a healthy weight. Within that calorie range, try to pick foods with a low percentage of fat, saturated fat, cholesterol, and sodium, and aim for the 100 percent of the daily value – again, in your calorie range – of total carbohydrates and fiber.

- **Vitamins and minerals.** If you have been diagnosed with a liver disease, talk with your physician about which vitamins and minerals you should incorporate into your diet, and which ones you should eliminate. (For instance, excessive iron consumption can be harmful for many liver patients.) Take special notice of the vitamin and mineral counts for those substances, and consult your doctor before you take daily vitamins and other nutritional supplements.

Unless you're at home in your kitchen, it is usually not possible to measure an exact proportion. If you stop at the local ice-cream stand after work on a hot day, how can you measure a half-cup serving? Or, in an Italian restaurant, how can you possibly know when you've eaten your half-cup portion of pasta?

In those instances, it helps to compare the servings to familiar objects. You may have to use your imagination, but with a little practice, you can make a fair guess as to how much you're really eating. Some common serving sizes and their comparative objects are as follows:

Serving Size	Object of Comparison
1 cup of cereal	a fist
1/2 cup cooked rice, pasta, or potato	half a baseball
1 "normal-sized" baked potato	a fist
1 medium fruit	a baseball
1/2 cup fresh fruit	half a baseball
1 1/2 ounces low-fat or fat-free cheese	4 stacked dice
1/2 cup ice cream	half a baseball
2 tablespoons peanut butter	a ping-pong ball

WEIGHT LOSS: A WEALTH OF OPTIONS

No one is going to say losing weight is easy. Choosing healthy foods can be confusing, and maintaining an exercise regimen takes commitment and discipline.

The good news is that today we can choose from an array of popular weight-loss plans. Some cost no money, while others charge a fee for membership or for the food involved in the plan. (Look at it as an investment in your future.)

Here are four of the most popular weight-loss programs promoted today, with brief notes comparing the essence of the programs. We offer no recommendations as to which is the most effective – in fact, we believe each one can be effective and safe for individuals who are overweight. No matter which program you choose to follow (from these or the many others available), exercise is absolutely essential to success in weight reduction and maintenance.

Before you start any diet-and-exercise plan, be sure to discuss it with your doctor.

- **The Atkins Diet.** It sounds like a dream: burgers loaded with bacon and melted cheese, creamy soups made with butter, sausage whenever you like. But thousands of people have lost tons of weight, literally, following this high-fat, low-carbohydrate diet. It is not for everyone; that juicy burger comes without a bun. Followers of the Atkins diet are real believers, but liver or heart patients should talk with their doctors about the amounts of protein and fat they would be eating on this diet, and the possible consequences. The diet plan in the book *Dr. Atkins' New Diet Revolution* (Avon Books, 2002) must be strictly adhered to; overconsumption of the meats and other fatty foods can bring weight gain, rather than loss. Go to www.atkins.com for more information.

- **Jenny Craig.** Since 1985, the Jenny Craig weight-loss program has promoted its eating plan based on small, frequent portions, coupled with moderate activity and a balanced life – the program's three-pronged approach to weight loss and healthy living. Participants in Jenny Craig purchase their specially prepared meals directly from the program; some plans vary with weekends "off." Meals are calorie-based and reflect the latest USDA food guidelines, emphasizing fresh fruits and vegetables, and whole grains. The price of meals includes access to a 24-hour help line. Go to www.jennycraig.com for more information.

- **The South Beach Diet.** Like the Atkins diet, South Beach was created by a medical doctor, restricts carbohydrates, and is available in a book. On this diet, no bread, potatoes, fruit, cereal, rice, pasta, carrots, or corn are permitted for the first two weeks, and their consumption is discouraged later. South Beach differs from the Atkins diet in that it distinguishes between "unhealthy" and "healthy" fats, and enthusiastically promotes the latter. Also, rather than counting grams of carbohydrates, the South Beach diet is based on a low glycemic index – i.e., a low amount of sugar in the carbohydrates – in a way that will remind some readers of the old Sugar Busters diet. Go to www.southbeachdiet.com for more information.

- **Weight Watchers.** Millions of men and women have lost weight with Weight Watchers since the program began in the early 1960s. All foods are permitted – one of the plan's biggest selling points – but the amount is restricted through a "points" plan; participants are told they will lose weight if their eating stays below a certain number of points each day, calculated according to their age, weight, and other factors. (A homemade éclair is 6 points; an ear of corn is 1 point; a 4-ounce glass of wine is 2 points, and so forth.) Members attend weekly meetings, are weighed periodically, and are encouraged to exercise. There is a weekly or monthly membership fee. Go to www.weightwatchers.com for more information.

DON'T SKIP YOUR MORNING COFFEE

Forget what you've heard about the hazards of being a coffee drinker. The latest research shows that not only does coffee deliver an abundance of antioxidants – packing more antioxidants, in fact, than blueberries or broccoli – but it also can reduce one's risk of chronic liver disease, particularly hepatocellular carcinoma (HCC), or primary liver cancer.

We already knew that a lunchtime latte helps us perk up in the afternoon. Athletes have long relied on caffeine to aid fatigued muscles and give them a slight edge in speed and endurance. These benefits probably are linked to coffee's ability to trigger an adrenaline release in our systems.

What is unexpected is the notion that coffee brings long-term benefits, including a mild antidepressant and inhibition of diabetes and even Parkinson's disease. Yet the findings are consistent in studies across the globe. For those at risk of liver disease, the good news is

WHAT'S YOUR DISEASE QUOTIENT?

Almost everyone's heritage brings risks of diseases. Arthritis might run in some families, while others carry a tendency toward heart disease or certain cancers. Now a new website will help you pinpoint your family's disease risk – and, even better, it will give you a targeted plan for lifestyle changes that can help you lower those genetic risks.

Developed by the Harvard Center for Cancer Prevention, the website www.yourdiseaserisk.com helps visitors calculate their risk of heart disease, diabetes, stroke, osteoporosis, and 12 different cancers. It not only employs the usual questions, such as age and family history, but also examines one's lifestyle choices, environment, and other factors. You will be shown a graphic that compares your risk to that of your fellow human beings. Then the real bonus appears: a specific, step-by-step plan – including recommended diet changes, exercise, and alcohol consumption – designed to lower your risks. And if you're not sure whether you want to skip that third glass of wine or run the extra 10 minutes, you can click on each step and see how that one action would change your disease risk.

that coffee can help prevent cirrhosis, liver cancer, and other serious chronic liver diseases.

At this writing, researchers have not pinpointed whether coffee's disease-preventive qualities are due to its dense antioxidants or to the caffeine itself. But the reduction in disease risk, including a diminished risk of developing liver cancer, is solidly supported by evidence: As little as two cups of coffee a day can help protect an at-risk patient from developing a more serious liver disease.

It is still true that some coffee drinkers experience "the jitters" or an upset stomach. If coffee causes you physical discomfort or keeps you awake at night, you probably should use it only in moderation, and pregnant women are advised to avoid excessive caffeine. Other than those caveats, the biggest danger from coffee use appears to be the extra calories we add when we load it with sugar and whipped cream.

GET MOVING!

Diet alone won't keep us healthy. Most people can recite the benefits of regular exercise – weight control, lower anxiety levels, better concentration, higher self-esteem, good balance, and chronic-pain management, to name just a few – but knowing, of course, isn't enough.

When 17,000 fitness professionals certified by the American Council on Exercise (ACE) were asked to name the one exercise they couldn't live without, the runaway winner was the multi-purpose squat. That one movement strengthens every major muscle below the waist – gluteals, hamstrings, quadriceps, and calves. The respondents' top choices:

- Squats
- Running
- Abdominal exercise
- Lunges
- Walking
- Push-ups
- Yoga

Today, we know that one of the most damaging places to carry extra weight is in the belly. Older women, though, have one advantage in trimming down ab flab, even if they are genetically predisposed to acquiring it: resistance training. A University of Alabama study of men and women ages 61 to 77 years showed that, after 25 weeks of resistance training three times a week, both men and women improved their strength equally and lost about 4.4 pounds of total body fat – but the women lost theirs from their abdomens.

With exercise requirements as with nutrition, the USDA has stepped up to provide guidelines. They define physical activity simply as body movement that uses energy. They recommend 30 minutes of moderate exercise each day to maintain good health, though more vigorous or sustained exercise might be needed for weight loss. Examples of moderate activities include brisk walking (three and a half miles per hour), hiking, gardening or yard work, dancing, golf (walking and carrying clubs), bicycling (less than 10 miles per hour), and general, light weight training.

For vigorous activities, the USDA includes running or jogging (five miles per hour), bicycling (more than 10 miles per hour), swimming, aerobics, and fast walking (four and a half miles per hour), among other more strenuous activities that may not always be suitable for older people.

KEEPING FIT ON THE ROAD

Travel is exhausting, physically and emotionally, under the best of circumstances, and everyone – especially those with chronic illnesses, such as a liver disease – needs to keep wellness goals in mind while traveling. Eating the wrong foods, drinking too much, and getting little exercise can drain you physically in only a few days. Instead, follow these easy tips for staying healthy on the go:

- You can always exercise. If there are no parks or trails nearby, every hotel has a staircase and corridors for walking – but why not head outdoors and explore the neighborhood for an hour? Many destinations offer maps of self-guided walking tours, or you can easily devise your own.

- Be sure to carry comfortable walking shoes when you travel, along with the right socks and a lightweight outfit for exercise.

- Carry exercise bands in your suitcase – a lightweight way to do resistance exercises in your hotel room.

- Don't skip meals when you travel; it is too easy to become famished and overeat at dinner. Carry high-nutrient, high-fiber, low-sugar nutrition bars; they're handy when you don't want to stop for a full meal.

- Drink plenty of bottled water whenever you travel. One 8-ounce glass per hour during flight is a good standard.

- On long flights, get up for a few minutes every hour or so. Stand on your toes, roll back on your heels – exercise those lower-body muscles a bit. Back in your seat, perform some sitting exercises. (Check the seat pockets: Most airlines now provide cards with suggested moves.)

(continued on page 179)

IF YOU NEED HELP

If you abuse alcohol or smoke any cigarettes at all, these resources will help you conquer your problem:

FOR SMOKERS

www.smokefree.gov. This site offers an easy-to-read online guide to quitting tobacco for good, starting with specific steps to take on "quit day." It also provides reasons to quit, tips for sticking with it, studies, and other useful information.

www.cancer.org, (800) ACS-2345. Along with basic quitting techniques, the American Cancer Society's site offers tips for avoiding weight gain, stress, and withdrawal symptoms, and for handling maintenance.

www.cdc.gov/tobacco/quit_smoking/index.htm, (800) QUIT-NOW. The Centers for Disease Control's site makes smokers aware of immediate (and long-term) benefits of quitting, techniques for stopping tobacco, youth-oriented prevention programs, and information on secondhand smoke and other topics.

FOR ALCOHOL ABUSERS

www.alcoholics-anonymous.org. AA is a hugely successful program, with more than 2 million members in 150 countries. Learn about this meeting-based group and its 12-Step Recovery program, and get information on abstinence and how to find a meeting near you.

www.WebMD.com/mental-health/Alcohol-Abuse. WebMD.com is a popular health-information resource for consumers. This section outlines how to tell whether you have a drinking problem, offers tips on quitting alcohol today, and provides a variety of other resources.

www.collegedrinkingprevention.gov. For students, parents, and teachers, this site gives the facts about alcohol poisoning, along with tips on cutting alcohol use and other information.

- To avoid becoming dehydrated and fatigued, watch your alcohol and caffeine intake when you fly.

- In a new time zone, get some sunshine and try to stay awake the first day until bedtime without napping.

- Enjoy the local cuisine. Taste everything that pleases you, but fill up on healthier foods such as cooked vegetables and brown rice. ◆

Chapter 18

Looking Toward the Future

In many ways, the future is bright. Researchers are making promising advances in their understanding of disorders of the liver, and research progress is leading to new treatments for all forms of chronic liver disease. In addition to the new research, liver transplantation is becoming increasingly accessible, and we are seeing better long-term outcomes. Most people can expect to find a treatment approach to any form of liver disease they may acquire or develop. And if treatment is not successful, liver transplantation is usually available.

Another bright spot in the world of liver disease is the decline in new cases of chronic viral hepatitis. This global trend has developed for a number of reasons. Vaccines for chronic hepatitis B are extremely effective and will, we hope, lead to a worldwide eradication of this disease. Also, both lay and medical personnel now have a heightened awareness of the need for education and safety in the handling of blood and body fluids. Increased safety measures are also observed in connection with blood transfusions, which have been improved by developments in testing procedures that go back to the early 1990s.

One aspect of liver disease is showing an upsurge: NAFLD/NASH. This increase in nonalcoholic fatty liver disease and nonalcoholic steatohepatitis parallels the spread of the diabetes and obesity epidemic raging in America and throughout the world. But this story, too, has a silver lining. Researchers are investigating a variety of medications that show promise for the prevention and treatment of these conditions.

Science and technology are advancing rapidly and so are our successes against these diseases. However, there is still much work to do and there are many patients to care for. We hope that everyone reading this book will consider these facts if the opportunity to participate in a clinical trial arises. With solid research and motivated patients, we can work together to find new treatments or cures that will help our patients live long and happy lives. ◆

Appendix A

DRUG-INDUCED LIVER INJURY

The cut on Howie Elgin's leg wasn't the first he had received working as a tree cutter for the city. Nor did it seem that serious; it was more of a bad scrape than a cut. He had tripped over a section of tree branch, and as he fell, the bark had chafed the inside of his lower leg. There hadn't even been much bleeding.

Howie was only mildly concerned when the scrape became infected. As soon as he noticed swelling in that part of his leg, he went to the city's health-care provider, where the doctor prescribed amoxicillin-clavulanate, a popular antibiotic commonly known by its brand name of Augmentin.

The injury seemed to clear up quickly. Howie never felt much pain, and he didn't miss more than a few hours of work. By that weekend, though, he wasn't feeling well. His upper abdomen ached and by Sunday, he was somewhat nauseated. But he told himself it was "flu season" and he went to work the following week as usual.

Only when a co-worker mentioned that he "looked a little yellow" did Howie become alarmed. That evening, he asked his girlfriend whether she thought he "looked jaundiced." After one close look at his eyes and skin, she agreed: They showed a definite yellowish tint. At that point, Howie didn't want to waste another moment, and his girlfriend drove him to the closest hospital.

Howie suspected that something bad was happening to his liver, since jaundice is so closely associated with liver disease, and he was right. But he was amazed to learn that the damage was caused not by his infection, but by the cure! His Augmentin had triggered a drug-induced liver injury (DILI), an uncommon but not unheard-of reaction to certain prescription medications. In Howie's case, the remedy for his DILI was straightforward: He stopped taking the Augmentin. Over the next several weeks his liver tests showed quick improvement, and his skin tone returned to its normal color.

DIAGNOSING DRUG-INDUCED LIVER INJURY

Drug-induced liver injury (DILI) seems counterintuitive. DILI refers to a liver-test abnormality caused by the use of a specific medication – in other words, it is as if the patient came down with an illness that was caused by a cure. It is a common occurrence and one that is not always easy to diagnose or confirm. There are no lab tests one can order to determine that a specific medication actually caused the liver injury or the elevation in liver tests. In fact, many other conditions can mimic drug-induced liver injury and may need to be excluded before a diagnosis can be made. What's more, the medication that triggers the DILI usually was prescribed for a condition totally unrelated to liver disease, such as high blood pressure or a bacterial infection. A comprehensive history and a few routine laboratory tests usually are the best means of deciphering the clues and identifying the culprit.

Not only is DILI common, but it also has a broad spectrum in terms of clinical presentation – that is, symptoms and test results – ranging from mild elevations in ALT/AST enzymes to a much more severe injury leading to jaundice and at times liver failure. (See the table at the end of this section.) And, the diagnosed ailment might closely resemble a different disease altogether; a number of drugs have been implicated as causes of a chronic hepatitis syndrome that can be indistinguishable from autoimmune hepatitis. The result can be that a patient is placed on corticosteroids instead of taken off the offending agent. This can obviously lead to further problems connected with use of oral corticosteroids and further use of the offending agent. Commonly prescribed medications that have been shown to cause this condition include minocycline, nitrofurantoin, and methyldopa.

One unique form of drug-induced liver toxicity is connected with methotrexate, which may cause liver fibrosis or scarring after being taken for long periods of time. This medication is now most commonly used to treat rheumatoid arthritis and related autoimmune problems. It is also frequently used by dermatologists to treat refractory psoriasis. After it has been used for long periods, a "cumulative dose" exposure is often calculated. If this dose is high enough or the liver lab tests look abnormal, a liver biopsy may be obtained. The good news is that the lower doses of methotrexate currently used do not appear to be as damaging to the liver as was once thought. (To all patients taking methotrexate: Please do not stop this medication unless you discuss it with your physician first.)

Another rare side effect of medications is drug-induced liver tumors. This particular complication has been linked to the use of oral contraceptive pills in women of childbearing age. These women may develop benign tumors termed adenomas. In rare cases, the tumor could be malignant.

In general, once the offending medication in a DILI is removed, liver tests will improve and normalize over the following weeks. This can be highly variable, though, depending on the medication and its

PHARMACOGENOMICS AND PHAMACOGENETICS

A new approach to testing for a patient's susceptibility to DILI is emerging. This new approach is known as pharmacogenomics or pharmacogenetics. The terms can be used interchangeably and basically refer to the study of variations in a patient's DNA as it relates to a drug response. This emerging area of study can help determine whether a patient will respond to or resist a specific medication. At present these tests have limited availability. Hopefully, as research continues, lab tests will become available to assist the clinician in tailoring a medication treatment plan to each individual. In time this may also mean that unnecessary toxicity can be avoided simply through analysis of the individual's DNA.

active metabolites. For some medications there will be continued abnormalities for weeks to months after the offending medication is withdrawn. It is rare for patients to be exposed intentionally to the offending medication in order to establish the diagnosis. This should absolutely not be tried if a patient developed jaundice during the initial DILI. For the rare or special circumstance when a diagnosis is in question a liver biopsy may be obtained.

COMMON MEDICATIONS ASSOCIATED WITH LIVER INJURY

The following familiar medications are known to react on livers:

Acetaminophen (Tylenol). Acetaminophen is the most common cause of acute liver failure in the United States. The recommended dose on most bottles indicates that a person should not exceed 4 grams in a day (8 tablets of extra-strength Tylenol). This dosage is generally safe and effective for most people. This is *not* true, though, for persons regularly using or abusing alcohol. For people who regularly use and or abuse alcohol, even a lower dose of acetaminophen may cause significant liver injury.

When a patient accidentally or intentionally ingests a toxic dose of acetaminophen, treatment is indicated. A toxic dose is generally regarded as more than 10 to 15 grams (20 to 30 extra-strength tablets or capsules) of acetaminophen in a 24-hour period. Treatment usually includes hospitalization and treatment with N-acetylcysteine, otherwise referred to as NAC. Most patients improve and are released without long-term problems. However, a small number of these patients will progress to acute liver failure and require a liver transplant.

Amoxicillin-clavulanate (Augmentin). This antibiotic has been used clinically for more than two decades to treat numerous types of bacterial infections. It also has been implicated as one of the most common causes of DILI worldwide.

The type and severity of injury that develops is quite variable. Amoxicillin-clavulanate-related DILI may develop during or shortly after completion of the course of treatment, but most drug-induced liver injuries are mild and self-limited, even for patients who develop jaundice. There have been rare instances in which a patient develops severe hepatotoxicity and requires a liver transplant. Again, these severe reactions are extremely rare. This medication has been used extensively and safely for decades.

Isoniazid or INH (Nydrazid). Anyone taking this medication (usually given for the treatment of tuberculosis) should be concerned about the potential for hepatotoxicity. In fact, 10 percent to 20 percent of patients taking INH will develop a mild degree of AST/ALT elevation. These elevations usually start at the beginning of treatment and are frequently noted, since lab monitoring for liver toxicity is recommended. Fortunately, most patients who develop mild liver-enzyme elevations will adapt to the medication and the enzymes will return to normal even when the medication is continued. It has been estimated that only about 1 percent of patients over age 50 will develop significant liver injury while undergoing treatment, especially if this treatment is combined with other medications used to treat tuberculosis, such as rifampin or pyrazinamide. Other variables that may increase a patient's risk of developing drug-induced liver injury include alcohol abuse, chronic hepatitis B, chronic hepatitis C, or HIV infection.

Minocycline (Minocin or Dynacin). Thousands of people across the country take minocycline on a daily basis to treat acne. Most people take this medication without any problem or experience of toxicity. Unfortunately, this drug also has been shown to cause several different types of hepatotoxicity. The most striking reaction occurs when a chronic hepatitis develops that mimics chronic autoimmune hepatitis. Most patients who develop this condition are young people who have taken the medication for months without a problem. As mentioned before, a hepatologist should be consulted for cases when someone taking minocycline suddenly develops or is diagnosed with autoimmune hepatitis. The consultation is crucial, as both treatment and nontreatment can lead to further problems if not managed appropriately.

Lipid-lowering agents or statins (Lipitor, Zocor, Crestor). Collectively called statins, this common class of medications is used to treat elevated cholesterol and triglycerides. Statins work in similar ways but may have differing degrees of potency. These medications have received extensive attention because they are widely used and have a propensity to cause elevations in liver enzymes (AST/ALT). It is estimated that 1 percent to 3 percent of patients on statins will develop significantly elevated enzymes (greater than three times the upper limit of normal).

As the treatment guidelines for lowering cholesterol have become more aggressive, the number of people taking these medications has increased substantially over the past decade, leaving many clinicians (usually primary care providers) unclear about whether these medications should be used in patients with underlying liver disease and when to stop if liver enzymes become abnormal. While these questions have not been fully answered, statins seem extremely safe and should not be avoided by patients with underlying liver diseases if the statins are indicated for the treatment of high cholesterol or triglycerides. (The benefits outweigh the risks.)

Most patients who develop an increase in liver enzymes during therapy with statins will have only transient and mild elevation, which will subsequently resolve if the medication is stopped.

Ezetimibe (Zetia). This is another cholesterol-lowering medication, but it is not in the statin class of drugs. In fact, it is frequently used with a statin when cholesterol cannot be lowered by the statin alone. This medication works by inhibiting the intestinal uptake of cholesterol. In extremely rare cases reports have connected it with drug-induced liver injury, but it is regarded as having an excellent safety profile. However, it is currently undergoing reevaluation of its effectiveness in preventing heart disease and stroke. ◆

CAUSES OF DRUG-INDUCED LIVER INJURY

Category	Examples	Typical Indication or Use
Elevated transaminases (ALT or AST) (Drug-induced hepatitis)	Variety of antibiotics Isoniazid Statins Amiodarone Aspirin Nitrofurantoin Phenytoin Alcohol	Infection Tuberculosis Elevated cholesterol Heart disorders Blood-thinner Urinary tract infection Seizures No indication
Elevated alkaline phosphatase and/or bilirubin (Drug-induced cholestasis and jaundice)	Amoxicillin-clavulanate Erythromycin	Infection Infection
Fatty liver (Drug-induced steatosis)	Tetracycline Valproic acid Alcohol Corticosteroids Amiodarone	Acne Seizures No indication Anti-inflammatory Heart disorders
Liver failure (Drug-induced liver failure)	Acetaminophen Mushroom poisoning Halothane Isoniazid Nonsteroidal anti-inflammatory drugs	Pain No indication Anesthesia Tuberculosis Pain or inflammation
Liver scarring (Drug-induced fibrosis)	Methotrexate	Rheumatoid arthritis, psoriasis
Tumors (Drug-induced hepatic tumors)	Oral contraceptives Anabolic steroids	Birth control Muscle building

COMMON LIVER-RELATED TERMINOLOGY

Acute alcoholic hepatitis: An acute hepatitis that is sometimes caused by chronic, heavy alcohol ingestion.

Alpha fetoprotein (AFP) test: A biochemical blood test that can help in detecting liver cancer.

Albumin: A protein manufactured by the liver. Low albumin levels in the blood usually indicate poor liver function, but may also reflect poor nutrition and disease of other organs (e.g., kidneys).

Alcoholic liver disease: Liver disease caused by excessive consumption of alcohol. The damage can range from too much fat in the liver to cirrhosis or liver failure.

Alkaline phosphatase test: A lab test that measures a protein found in bile-duct cells. Blood levels may increase in any liver disease, but the elevation is more marked with a problem involving bile flow.

ALT (alanine aminotransferase, also known as alanine transaminase) test: A lab test that measures an enzyme that is increased when liver cells (hepatocytes) show increased activity or are damaged.

Aminotransferase enzymes: Alanine aminotransferase (ALT) and aspartate aminotransferase (AST); sometimes called transaminases.

Anemia: A condition in which the blood is deficient in oxygen-carrying red blood cells.

Antimitochondrial antibody test: A lab test used in the diagnosis of primary biliary cirrhosis.

Antinuclear antibody test: When this lab test has a positive result, it suggests that some type of autoimmune illness may be present.

Ascites: An accumulation of fluid in the abdominal cavity. This occurs when the blood flow through the liver is obstructed. Ascites most commonly occurs as a secondary condition when cirrhosis is present.

AST (aspartate aminotransferase, also known as aspartate transaminase) test: A lab test measuring an enzyme that increases when liver cells (hepatocytes) show increased activity or are damaged. It is not as specific as the ALT for liver injury.

Asterixis (liver flap): An uncontrollable flapping of the outstretched hands sometimes seen in cases of advanced liver disease; it is related to encephalopathy.

Autoimmune disorder: Occurs when a person's immune system attacks itself as if it were a foreign invader.

Autoimmune hepatitis: A form of chronic hepatitis that occurs when the body's immune system attacks its own liver.

Azathioprine (Imuran): A drug generally used to treat autoimmune diseases. It is most commonly used both with and without prednisone to treat autoimmune hepatitis.

Bile: A yellow-green fluid produces in the liver and stored in the gallbladder. Bile helps the body break down fats and digest fat-soluble vitamins.

Bile duct: A large tubelike structure through which bile travels from the liver to the small intestine.

Biliary atresia: A congenital condition in which bile from the liver cannot reach the intestine because the bile ducts are not developed properly.

Bilirubin: The breakdown product of old red blood cells. This product is excreted by the liver; normally it is excreted in the bile. If the bilirubin is not properly excreted, the serum bilirubin rises and leads to jaundice.

Blood pressure: The pressure of blood in the arteries. The top number is the systolic pressure; it refers to blood pressure when the heart is contracting. The lower number is the diastolic pressure; it refers to when the heart muscle is relaxed.

Blood products: A general term for different compounds of blood that can be transfused into patients, such as packed red blood cells or platelets and concentrated clotting proteins used for treating people with hemophilia.

Bone marrow: The soft tissue inside the bones, where red and white blood cells and platelets are made.

Caput medusae: Literally "Medusa's head," it means dilated varicose veins around the umbilicus that may be seen in patients with cirrhosis.

Ceruloplasmin: A copper-containing protein; blood tests usually show decreased levels in Wilson disease.

Cholangiocarcinoma: A cancer that starts in the bile ducts or biliary tree.

Cholestasis: Failure of bile to flow from the liver through the bile ducts and into the small intestine.

Chronic viral hepatitis: Chronic infection of the liver, resulting from the hepatitis viruses B and C, that persists for longer than six months.

Cirrhosis: A term used to describe extensive scarring or fibrosis of the liver. Under a microscope the scar tissue or fibrosis is said to contain "regenerative nodules."

Clotting factors: Substances made mainly in the liver that help the blod clot normally. Declining liver function results in a decreased clotting ability. Patients with liver disease often have excessive bleeding. A lack of clotting factors is one of the reasons for this.

Coagulopathy: A tendency for increased bleeding due to decreased hepatic synthesis of clotting factors. It is usually a sign of advanced liver disease.

Complete early virologic response (cEVR): Term for the patient's recovery when no virus or "viral load" is detected after 12 weeks of pegylated interferon therapy for chronic HCV.

Computerized tomography (CT) scan: A specialized x-ray procedure that uses computers to construct a two-dimensional picture of the body or, more specifically, of the liver.

Corticosteroids: Drugs that suppress inflammation throughout a person's body. Common names include prednisolone, prednisone, and hydrocortisone.

Creatinine test: A lab test that measures a product of muscle metabolism that is excreted by the kidneys. The creatinine level is used to assess kidney function.

Cryptogenic: Literally means "unknown cause." Sometimes liver fibrosis or cirrhosis occurs, but no known cause can be identified. The term "cryptogenic cirrhosis" is used to distinguish it from other known causes of cirrhosis such as hepatitis C or alcohol-induced cirrhosis.

Cyclosporin A (Sandimmune and Neoral): A chemotherapeutic agent given to organ-transplant recipients to prevent the body from rejecting the new organ.

Doppler ultrasound of the liver, or liver vascular ultrasound: A painless test using sound waves to show whether or not the blood flow to and from the liver is normal.

Early virologic response (EVR): Defined as a viral load reduction greater than two logs from baseline after initiation of pegylated interferon treatment for chronic HCV. This is further divided into partial early viral response (pEVR) and complete early viral response (cEVR). (See separate definitions for each.)

Electrolytes: Minerals present in a person's body fluids that are frequently altered with diuretics. Common electrolytes are: sodium, potassium, chloride, magnesium, and calcium.

Endoscope: A flexible instrument used to examine the esophagus, stomach, and duodenum. When found by endoscope, varices of the esophagus can be banded or ligated.

Encephalopathy: An alteration in mental status, ranging from forgetfulness and mild confusion to coma. It may be caused by circulating, gut-derived, brain-toxic byproducts not cleared by a dysfunctional liver.

ERCP test: Endoscopic retrograde cholangio pancreatography. A special test using an endoscope to examine the bile ducts or biliary tree.

Esophageal varices: Dilated blood vessels in the esophagus that usually result from portal hypertension (a high-pressure state behind the liver, secondary to cirrhosis). Varices can rupture and cause a life-threatening upper GI bleed.

Esophagus: The tube between the mouth and stomach through which food and liquids pass.

Fatty liver: Excessive deposition of fat in the liver. A liver has to be at least 30 percent fat for the deposit to be noted on imaging such as an ultrasound or a CT scan.

Ferritin: A lab test that measures an iron-containing serum protein in the blood. This test is used to monitor the effects of deironization in patients with hemochromatosis.

Fibrosis: The formation of fibrous tissue, or scarring.

Gallbladder: A reservoir that stores bile secreted by the liver. The gallbladder empties the bile into the intestine to help with digestion.

Gallstones: "Stones" that form in the gallbladder and are usually composed mainly of cholesterol. They can lead to gallstone colic (pain due to blockage of the gallbladder outlet), cholecystitis (inflammation of the gallbladder), and possibly jaundice if they move out of the gallbladder and block the bile ducts.

Gastroenterologist: A physician who specializes in treating diseases of the digestive system and liver.

GGTP (gamma-glutamyl transpeptidase) test: A lab test that measures an enzyme synthesized by the liver. High levels can sometimes be seen when there is obstruction of bile flow. The test is very nonspecific.

Graft: When a new organ is transplanted, the transplant is referred to as a graft.

Hemochromatosis: Sometimes referred to as "bronze diabetes." A genetic disorder that causes increased absorption of iron by the gastrointestinal tract. The iron can accumulate in the liver and lead to cirrhosis. Increased iron can also cause heart problems, diabetes, and arthritis.

Hepatic: Referring to the liver.

Hepatic artery: The main artery that supplies oxygenated blood to the liver.

Hepatic vein: The vein that drains blood from the liver toward the heart.

Hepatitis: A general term used to describe any inflammation of the liver.

Hepatitis A: An acute viral hepatitis caused by the hepatitis A virus. There is no chronic form. It usually resolves in a few weeks and is rarely fatal. It is transmitted by contaminated food and water.

Hepatitis B: A viral hepatitis caused by the hepatitis B virus. It is transmitted by blood or body fluids. Full recovery occurs in more than 90 percent of individuals infected as adults. Chronic hepatitis B can lead to cirrhosis and is most commonly found in Asia.

Hepatitis C: A viral hepatitis caused by the hepatitis C virus. It is most commonly transmitted by infected blood. Individuals may develop chronic hepatitis, which can lead to cirrhosis and liver failure.

Hepatitis D: A viral particle that infects individuals only when they are already infected with hepatitis B. When found, it usually is associated with more severe liver disease.

Hepatitis E: A viral hepatitis caused by the hepatitis E virus. It is transmitted by infected food and water. It is rarely seen in the United States. It carries a significant risk of fatality in pregnant women.

Hepatocellular carcinoma (HCC): A primary liver tumor more common in patients with cirrhosis.

Hepatocytes: Liver cells.

Hepatologist: A physician who specializes in liver diseases and the treatment of patients before and after a liver transplant.

Immunosuppressive medications: Drugs that suppress the body's immune system. They are used to help prevent the organ recipient from rejecting the new organ.

Inflammatory bowel disease (IBD): Most commonly ulcerative colitis and Crohn's disease. They are often associated with sclerosing cholangitis.

Interferon, pegylated (Pegasys, Peg-Intron): Immunomodulator drugs used to treat hepatitis B and C. Interferons are natural substances produced by the body that help to enhance the immune system.

Jaundice: A yellowish color affecting the eyes and skin that is due to excess bilirubin in the blood. Jaundice usually occurs because the liver fails to excrete bilirubin in the normal manner. It also results from liver failure or obstruction in the biliary tree.

Kayser-Fleischer rings: Golden-brown rings seen in slit-lamp examination of the cornea; they result from copper deposition in Wilson disease.

Lipids: A general term for cholesterol and triglycerides in the blood.

Liver function tests (LFTs): A common panel of blood tests used to evaluate a person's liver. The LFTs usually include the bilirubin, AST, ALT, albumin, and alkaline phosphatase. This is sometimes referred to as a hepatic function panel or HFP.

Mycophenolate mofetil (Cellcept): A drug given to transplant recipients to prevent the body from rejecting the new organ.

Osteoporosis: A decrease in the density of bones that makes them more likely to fracture.

Partial early virologic response (pEVR): This is identified when a patient achieves a greater-than-two log reduction in HCV RNA "viral load" from baseline after 12 weeks of pegylated interferon therapy. Some quantifiable virus remains and can be detected. Therefore, it is referred to as partial response as opposed to complete response, with no virus detected.

Platelets: Cells in the blood that help it to clot. The platelet count usually decreases with cirrhosis as the platelets are stored in the enlarged spleen.

Portal hypertension: Increased pressure in the portal vein and blood vessels behind the liver, most commonly seen secondary to cirrhosis of the liver.

Portal vein: A large vein that carries blood from the intestines to the liver on its way to the heart.

Portosystemic encephalopathy (PSE): Another term for encephalopathy.

Primary biliary cirrhosis (PBC): A chronic cholestatic liver disease most commonly seen in women.

Primary sclerosing cholangitis (PSC): A progressive liver disorder that causes destruction of the bile ducts. Patients with PSC are frequently afflicted with inflammatory bowel disease.

Prophylaxis: The prevention of a problem. For example, beta blockers that are antihypertensive medications are often used to prevent esophageal varices from rupturing.

PT/INR (prothrombin time/international normalized ratio) test: A lab test that measures the time it takes for a blood sample to clot. The test can be a reflection of overall liver synthetic function.

Ribavirin (Copegus, Rebetol): A drug used in combination with interferon to treat viral hepatitis C because it makes interferon more effective.

Pruritus: Itching.

Rapid virologic response: Defined as a nondetectable HCV RNA after four weeks of pegylated interferon therapy for chronic HCV. This result is a very good indicator for treatment success.

Red blood cells: The blood cells that carry oxygen attached to hemoglobin.

Spider angiomas or nevi: Red capillary tufts in the skin that are supplied by a tiny artery and blanch upon pressure; often found in patients with chronic liver disease or cirrhosis.

Spleen: An organ that breaks down old blood cells. It becomes enlarged and sequesters (stores) platelets when a patient has cirrhosis with portal hypertension.

Spontaneous bacterial peritonitis (SBP): A bacterial infection of the ascitic fluid that occurs without a particular instigating incident or procedure.

Sustained virologic response (SVR): This is defined as the achievement of HCV RNA negativity six months after finishing a course of pegylated interferon therapy for chronic HCV.

Tacrolimus (Prograf): Previously known as FK506; a drug given to a transplant recipient to prevent the body from rejecting the new organ.

Thrombosis: The formation or presence of a blood clot.

Triglyceride: A type of body fat measured in a lipid panel. Elevated triglycerides are frequently seen in patients with diabetes or metabolic syndrome.

Viral load: The amount of a virus measured in 1 ml of blood. This lab test is usually measured in international units or IU's. Common examples include HCV RNA PCR quantitative or HBV DNA quantitative.

White blood cells: That part of the blood that fights infections.

Wilson disease: Inherited metabolic disorder in which copper accumulates in the liver and in the central nervous system, causing hepatitis, cirrhosis, and neuropsychiatric symptoms.

Appendix C

INDICATION	AGENT		
	BRAND NAME	GENERIC NAME	
Ascites	Aldactone Lasix Midamore	spironalactone furosemide amiloride	
Autoimmune hepatitis	Prednisone Imuran	prednisone azathioprine	
Cholestatic liver diseases	vitamins A,D,E,K	vitamins A,D,E,K	
Hepatic encephalopathy	Kristalose Flagyl Neomycin Xifaxan	lactulose metronidazole neomycin sulfate rifaximin	
Prevention of spontaneous bacterial peritonitis	Noroxin	norfloxacin	
Hepatitis C treatment	Pegasys Peg-Intron Copegus, Rebetol	pegylated interferon alpha 2a pegylated interferon alpha 2b ribavirin	
Hepatitis B treatment	Baraclude Epivir Tyzeka	entecavir lamivudine telbivudine	
Liver transplant	Cellcept Cyclosporin Prograf Rapamune	mycophenolate neoral tacrolimus sirolimus	
Prevention of bleeding from varices	Inderal Corgard	propranolol nadolol	
Primay biliary cirrhosis (PBC)	Actigall	ursodiol	
Primary sclerosing cholangitis (PSC)	Actigall, Urso	ursodiol	
Pruritus (itching)	Questran	cholestyramine	
Wilson disease	Cuprimine Syprine Orazinc	D-penicillamine trientine zinc sulfate	

MEDICATIONS COMMONLY USED IN LIVER DISEASE

DAILY DOSAGE RANGE	COMMON SIDE EFFECTS
25-400mg	Electrolyte abnormalities
20-160mg	Electrolyte abnormalities
5-20mg	Electrolyte abnormalities
1mg-60mg	Elevated glucose, fluid retention, mood swings
50-150mg	Bone-marrow suppression
per US-RDA guidelines	Usually none
10-40grams a day	Diarrhea
250-750mg	Metallic taste, headache, diarrhea; avoid with alcohol
500-1500mg	Diarrhea, kidney toxicity
200-600mg	Diarrhea
400mg	Phototoxicity, diarrhea
90-180mcg sq weekly	Nausea, muscle ache, fever, fatigue, depression, low white-cell count
80-150mcg sq weekly	Nausea, muscle ache, fever. fatigue, depression, low white- cell count
200-1200mg	Anemia, cough, skin rash
0.5-1.0mg	Headache, fatigue, nausea
100mg	Headache, fatigue, nausea
600mg	Headache, fatigue, nausea
500-1500mg	Diarrhea, hypertension, lipid abnormalities
25-200mg	Headache, glucose intolerance, kidney toxicity
0.5-10mg	Headache, glucose intolerance, kidney toxicity
1-10mg	Edema, impaired wound-healing, headache
30-240mg	Fatigue, hypotension, slow heart rate, decreased erectile function
20-320mg	Fatigue, hypotension, bradycardia
13-15mg/kg/day	Diarrhea, nausea, headache
15-21mg/kg/day	Diarrhea, nausea, headache
4-20grams	Gas, bloating, belching
250-1000mg	Neurological symptoms; allergic reaction, bone-marrow toxicity, lupuslike reaction
250-100mg	
110-220mg	Dizziness, diarrhea

Appendix D

SUGGESTED RESOURCES

The following websites and organizations will give you a good start toward learning more about your liver:

American Association for the Study of Liver Diseases
www.aasld.org
(703) 299-9766
AASLD exists mostly for physicians and liver researchers, but its staff can refer patients to a liver doctor.

American Gastroenterological Association
www.gastro.org
(301) 654-2055
Although the AGA's members are physicians and scientists, patients can use this website to find the latest research on liver diseases.

American Liver Foundation
www.liverfoundation.org
(800) GO-LIVER / (800) 465-4837
The premier national organization dedicated to promoting liver wellness and the prevention and treatment of liver diseases through research, education, and advocacy. Many chapters also sponsor support groups and seminars. For comprehensive information about your liver, the ALF is a good first stop.

Centers for Disease Control and Prevention
www.cdc.gov
(404) 639-3311
The CDC is a federal agency that provides updated health and medical information to consumers. To target your search, type the name of a specific illness (or simply "liver") into the search box.

Children's Liver Association for Support Services

www.classkids.org

(877) 679-8256

CLASS's mission is to provide emotional, educational, and financial support for families experiencing pediatric liver disease.

Cleveland Clinic Center for Continuing Education

www.clevelandclinicmeded.com

A comprehensive medical-information resource for health professionals. Among other information, you will find the following:

Hepatitis C Management

http://www.clevelandclinicmeded.com/online/monograph/HEPc/introduction.htm

Disease Management Project

(includes sections in hepatology)

http://www.clevelandclinicmeded.com/medicalpubs/disease management/gastroindex.htm

Cleveland Clinic Digestive Disease Center

(hepatology or liver section)

http://cms.clevelandclinic.org/digestivedisease/body.cfm?id=103

Hepatitis Foundation International

www.hepfi.org

(800) 891-0707

This is a major organization dedicated to hepatitis education, research, and treatment, and to the promotion of liver wellness.

HEP-C Connection

www.hepc-connection.org

(800) 522-4372

This organization provides support to families living with hepatitis C.

www.HIVandHepatitis.com

Designed for both patients and health-care professionals, this online magazine focuses on issues involved in HIV and hepatitis co-infection.

Latino Organization for Liver Awareness

www.lola-national.org

(888) 367-5652

LOLA is the first bilingual, bicultural, national organization to raise awareness of liver disease through referral services, educational outreach, and special events.

National Institutes of Health

www.nih.gov

(301) 496-1776

The NIH is a vast source of information on health and health research. Click on "Health," then "Health Topics A to Z" to find a wealth of information on liver wellness.

PBCers Organization

www.pbcers.org

This educational and support group is for patients diagnosed with primary biliary cirrhosis and other autoimmune liver diseases.

United Network for Organ Sharing

www.unos.org

(888) 894-6361

UNOS is the educational and scientific organization that administers the nation's Organ Procurement and Transplantation Network (OPTN). This is the site that will answer any question and respond to any concern connected with organ transplants and donation.

Veterans National Hepatitis C Program

www.hepatitis.va.gov

(877) 222-8387

This program gives health-care providers, veterans, and their families information about viral hepatitis.

Index

OTHER BOOKS FROM
CLEVELAND CLINIC PRESS

Age Well! A Cleveland Clinic Guide

Arthritis: A Cleveland Clinic Guide

Autopsy – Learning from the Dead: A Cleveland Clinic Guide

Battling the Beast Within: Success in Living with Adversity
(about multiple sclerosis)

Bladder Cancer: A Cleveland Clinic Guide

Breastless in the City: A Young Woman's Story of Love, Loss,
and Breast Cancer

Epilepsy – Information for You and Those Who Care About You:
A Cleveland Clinic Guide

Forever Home
(a chapter book for young readers)

Getting a Good Night's Sleep: A Cleveland Clinic Guide

The Granny-Nanny: A Guide for Parents and Grandparents
Who Share Child Care

Headaches: A Cleveland Clinic Handbook

Heart Attack: A Cleveland Clinic Guide

Heroes with a Thousand Faces: True Stories of People with Facial
Deformities and Their Quest for Acceptance

Lessons Learned: Stroke Recovery from a Caregiver's Perspective

My Grampy Can't Walk
   (a children's picture book about multiple sclerosis)

One Stroke, Two Survivors
   (the journey of a stroke victim and his wife)

Overcoming Infertility: A Cleveland Clinic Guide

Planting the Roses: A Cancer Survivor's Story
   (about esophageal cancer)

Prostate Cancer: A Cleveland Clinic Guide

Sober Celebrations: Lively Entertaining Without the Spirits
   (alcohol-free cooking)

Stop Smoking Now! The Rewarding Journey to a Smoke-Free Life

Tango: Lessons for Life
   (a dancing doctor's perspective on healing and life)

Thyroid Disorders: A Cleveland Clinic Guide

To Act As A Unit: The Story of the Cleveland Clinic
   (fourth edition)

Transplanting a Face: Notes on a Life in Medicine

Women's Health – Your Body, Your Hormones, Your Choices:
   A Cleveland Clinic Guide

Write for Life: Healing Body, Mind, and Spirit Through
   Journal Writing

You and Your Cardiologist: A Cleveland Clinic Guide

You CAN Eat That! Awesome Food for Kids with Diabetes

CLEVELAND CLINIC PRESS

Cleveland Clinic Press publishes nonfiction trade books for the medical, health, nutrition, cookbook, and children's markets. It is the mission of the Press to increase the health literacy of the American public and to dispel myths and misinformation about medicine, health care, and treatment. Our authors include leading authorities from Cleveland Clinic as well as a diverse list of experts drawn from medical and health institutions whose research and treatment breakthroughs have helped countless people.

Each Cleveland Clinic Guide provides the health-care consumer with practical and authoritative information. Every book is reviewed for accuracy and timeliness by Cleveland Clinic experts.

www.clevelandclinicpress.org

CLEVELAND CLINIC

Cleveland Clinic, located in Cleveland, Ohio, is a not-for-profit multispecialty academic medical center that integrates clinical and hospital care with research and education. Cleveland Clinic was founded in 1921 by four renowned physicians with a vision of providing outstanding patient care based upon the principles of cooperation, compassion, and innovation. *U.S. News & World Report* consistently names Cleveland Clinic as one of the nation's best hospitals in its annual "America's Best Hospitals" survey. Approximately 1,800 full-time salaried physicians at Cleveland Clinic and Cleveland Clinic Florida represent more than 120 medical specialties and subspecialties. In 2006, patients came for treatment from every state and 100 countries.

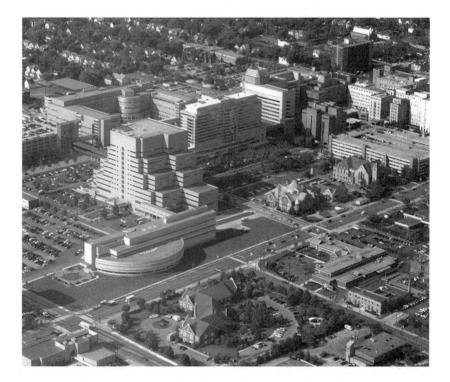

www.clevelandclinic.org